"Part Drucker, part Dyer, part Dilbert — *The Progress Challenge* is an entertaining and practical guide on how to achieve success in business and follow your bliss."

-- *Janet Gellici*
CEO, American Coal Council

"As friend, colleague and assistant to Dr. Viktor Frankl for over twenty years, I can confidently share with you that Dean Lindsay gets it! His ability to integrate the inspirational theories of Dr. Viktor Frankl with contemporary business needs is extraordinary. Dean's application of Frankl's concepts of "freedom of choice" and "the defiant power of the human spirit" to modern business/sales is powerfully motivating. *The Progress Challenge* goes beyond telling us to "just do it" and, in a very readable way, tells us how to do it - or, in Dean's words, how to be progress. A must read for business success!"

-- *Jay I. Levinson, Ph.D.*
Former Special Assistant to Dr. Viktor Frankl

"If you're serious about the Sales profession and Sales leadership, then this is the book for you. *The Progress Challenge* offers lots of helpful tips and ideas that will enhance your skills in the field of sales. Dean's style and sales examples keep you engaged throughout the book. This is a quick read and one that I enjoyed."

-- *Dave Nostrand*
Vice President, Sales - Eastern Region
Marriott International

"In a very engaging, fun and informative style, Dean Lindsay illuminates how, by redefining our views on change, we may all progress."

-- *Lusinè M. Meeks, GPHR*
Principal of Global Rewards and Mobility
Sabre Holdings

"If ever there was a right message at the right time, it's Dean Lindsay's book, *The Progress Challenge*. Dean is right that just changing isn't enough. We've got to make progress! Good ideas and practical examples."

-- Joe Calloway
Author, Becoming a Category of One

"Stop the management fads and the 'program of the month.' In *The Progress Challenge,* Dean Lindsay captures the issues and presents real, relevant, actionable solutions to the challenge of driving continual progress in business and life."

-- Tim McRay
Leadership and Diversity
Mercedes-Benz Financial

"Dean Lindsay has written a 'spot on' resourceful book! *The Progress Challenge* is a profound read that clearly speaks to seizing the time to effectively make progress, balancing through change, while void of stress and ultimately meeting and exceeding the challenge of becoming your best both personally and professionally."

-- Bradley D. Forsberg
Partner, KPMG

"*The Progress Challenge* offers leaders solutions and better tools for inspiring positive action. This is the first book on leadership that I have read from beginning to end without putting down. Dean Lindsay challenges, fascinates, and inspires the reader."

-- Jonas Milton (Stockholm, Sweden)
President (VD) of Almega

"Dean Lindsay is thinking big. Read this inspirational book and you will too."

-- Michael Port
Author, The Think Big Manifesto and Book Yourself Solid

"Personal responsibility and self-reliance are desperately needed today. These traits are what *The Progress Challenge* is about. Read Dean's book and savor the stories and seeds of thought that will help you to help those around you to be agents of...*Progress*, not just change. Don't just kick up dust; go out and make a difference."

-- Jim Cathcart
Author, Relationship Selling

"Outstanding! Dean Lindsay puts it all into perspective with *The Progress Challenge*. If you think your future is determined by fate, think again. Within these pages, Dean provides the questions and the encouragement that will help steer you into the future you desire and deserve. A 'makes you think' book for every leader and soon-to-be leader!"

-- Darrell Sims
Colonel, USAF (ret)

"This is a terrific and timely book with a simple but powerful message. With the right thinking and approach, we can make enormous progress in our organizations, with our families, and on our own goals and dreams. Dean's book shows you how, and provides the inspiration and advice you need to stay on track."

-- Brad Cleveland
Senior Advisor and Former President / CEO
International Customer Management Institute

"We all want our ideas, dreams, and plans to succeed. Dean Lindsay's *The Progress Challenge* is the perfect guidebook, providing the reader with understanding, motivation, support, and direction. Dean does all this with energy, humor and, most importantly, with thoughtfulness and care."

-- Joel Zeff
Author, Make the Right Choice

"When it's your time to make something great happen in your life or work, then this book is your answer. It contains a blueprint for reaching your personal best on a daily basis."
-- Mark LeBlanc
Author, Growing Your Business!

"Meeting the Progress Challenge will take your leadership and business to the next level. Dean Lindsay's book renews creativity and helps leaders remain focused on the critical elements of success, while navigating our ever-changing business world."
-- Bill Wallace
Chairman & CEO, The Wallace Companies
Founder, Success North Dallas

"Dean Lindsay writes like he speaks, with just the right mix of humor, thought-provoking concepts, and practical examples to make it a fun, easy, and valuable book to read. Whether you are in sales, marketing, or are a general business leader, you will walk away with a usable framework to positively deal with change, achieve progress, and immediately improve your results today!"
--Sean Piket
CEO, Sales Integrity and
Co-founder, SalesDiscipline.com

"*The Progress Challenge* makes a clear and valuable point that many people know what to do, but very few do what they know. As a sales leader for over 15 years, I have seen a lot of change in business. Dean does a great job in showing the difference and the benefits of Progress versus change."
-- Nathan Jamail
Author, The Sales Leaders Playbook

The Progress Challenge

The Progress Challenge

Working and Winning in a World of Change

Dean Lindsay
Progress Agent

The Progress Challenge Copyright © 2010 by Dean Lindsay.
Printed and bound in the United States of America. All Rights Reserved.

No part of this book may be used or reproduced in any manner whatsoever without written permission except in case of brief quotations embodied in critical articles and reviews. For information address: World Gumbo Publishing, 7801 Alma, Suite 105-323, Plano, TX 75025-3483

Although the author and publisher have made every effort to ensure the accuracy and completeness of information contained in this book, we assume no responsibility for errors, inaccuracies, omissions, or any inconsistency herein. The author and publisher specifically disclaim any responsibility for any liability, loss or risk, personal or otherwise, which is incurred as a consequence, directly or indirectly, of the use and application of any of the contents of this book. Any slights of people, places, or organizations are unintentional.

Paperback Edition 2011

LCCN: 2009932117

® Progress Agent, Be Progress and Six Ps of Progress are Registered Trademarks of Dean Lindsay

ATTENTION CORPORATIONS, UNIVERSITIES, COLLEGES, AND PROFESSIONAL ORGANIZATIONS:

Quantity discounts are available on bulk purchases of this book for educational, gift purposes, or as premiums for increasing magazine subscriptions or renewals. Special books or book excerpts can also be created to fit specific needs. For more information, please contact:
Info@WorldGumbo.com

Contact the Author at:
Dean@DeanLindsay.com
214-457-5656

To Jan Morgan
(My wonderful Mother)

Acknowledgments

Special Thanks to:
Doug Barkley, Jo-Ann Langseth, Dr. Bob Rich, Noel Mares, Martha Malnor, Cindy Peters, Dr. Jay Levinson, Vicki Snyder, Daren Martin, Robin Creasman, Scott Hasse, Devita Widmer, Jan Morgan, Shama Hyder, Malcolm Gilvar, Kristin Mapstone Smith, Marilyn and Tom Ross, Joy Jennings, Andra Grava, Nancy Barry, Russ McNeil, Lori Bourgo Lewis, Carolann Jacobs, Andra Grava, Robin Courtney, Jim Penny, Walter Nusbaum, Bill Wallace, Martha Lawrence, Renee Broadwell, Mark Washum, Jim Young, Sean Piket, Neil Shiller, Linda Boyle, Jeff Rhoades, Maria Smith, Lewis Dauria, Danell Winsor, Pat Dougher, Lori-Lynn Baker, Bob Schmidt, and to all the fine authors and business professionals who endorsed this project.

Extra Special Thanks to **Julie Weber.** *Having someone with your expertise – and in your position at such a fine organization – write the foreword to this book is just perfect. Thank you Julie.*

Extra Super Special Thanks to **Lena, Sofia & Ella** *-I love you.*

Credits:
Editor: Jo-Ann Langseth – Warwick, Rhode Island
Editorial Insight: Dr. Bob Rich – Healesville, Victoria (Australia)
Index: Martha Malnor – Katy, Texas
Cover Design & Layout: Noel Mares / The Trade Group – Carrolton, Texas with Dean Lindsay
Author Photo: Betsye Hamilton – Plano, Texas
Book Manufacturing: Thomson-Shore, Inc. – Dexter, Michigan

The Progress Challenge

> Challenge – *1. A call or summons to engage in any contest, as of skill, strength. 2. A demand to explain, justify. 3. Difficulty in a job or undertaking that is stimulating to one engaged in it. 4. Something that by its nature or character serves as a call for special effort.*

Contents

Foreword by Julie Weber   **11**
Senior Director, People, Southwest Airlines

To Change Is Human; to Progress, Divine.   13

The Way of the Donut Man   **15**

The Progress Challenge Revealed   **19**

To Change Is Human; to Progress, Divine   **23**
Ponder & Progress: Progress or Change?   *27*

Reasons Create Movement   **29**
Ponder & Progress: Reasons Create Movement   *32*

Becoming a Progress Agent   **33**
Ponder & Progress:
Uncovering Others' Parameters for Progress   *34*

The Rise of Progress Leadership –   **35**
    Change Management Is Dead
Super Quick Action Steps
to Excelling at Progress Leadership   *39*

Partnering to Progress   **41**
Ponder & Progress: Partnering to Progress   **44**

The Six Ps of Progress   45

The Progress Principle   47

Peace of Mind   53
The Way of Customer Care –
    Earning and Maintaining Customer Loyalty   55
Ponder & Progress: Defining Your Way
    of Customer Care   60
Ponder & Progress: The Peace of Mind 10   62

Pleasure   63
The Way of the Donut Man Revisited   67
Ponder & Progress: The Pleasure 10   69

Profit   71
The Way of a BAM –
    Becoming a Business Attraction Magnet   73
Seven Keys to Being a BAM   74
Ponder & Progress: Sales & Organization   79
Ponder & Progress: The Profit 10   83

Prestige   85
The Name Game   87
The Way of the Compliment   89
Ponder and Progress: The Prestige 10   91

Pain Avoidance   93
The Way of the Entrepreneurial Drill Sergeant   97
Ponder & Progress: The Pain Avoidance 10   102

Power   103
The Way of Viktor Frankl   107
Ponder & Progress: The Power 10   113

What About Pride and Purpose?   115

Progress in the Balance of Life 119
Life Is a Smorgasbord *121*
Ponder & Progress: A Life in the Balance *128*

Too Stressed to Progress *129*
Ponder & Progress: Too Stressed to Progress *133*
From Stress to Progress: Ten Tips *135*

Always Time to Progress *143*
Ponder & Progress: Always Time to Progress *144*
Always Time for Progress: Ten Tips *145*

Finding Progress in Change 153
Stop, BOP & Roll *155*
Stop *157*
BOP – Be Open to Progress *161*
Roll *165*
Ponder & Progress: Finding Progress in Change *168*

Committing to Progress 169
Don't Have to Do Anything, But Can't Do Nothing *171*
Defining Your Parameters for Progress *175*

An Introduction to Progress Based Goal-Crafting *179*
A Progress Agent's Six Rules for Goal-Crafting *181*

Committing to Progress *189*
Ponder & Progress: Committing to Progress *193*

Progress Takes Persistence *195*
Ponder & Progress: Progress Takes Persistence *201*

The Little Mind That Could 203

Index 207

About the Author 215

The Progress Challenge

Foreword by Julie Weber
Senior Director, People, Southwest Airlines

Let me just get this out first: *The Progress Challenge* is a great book. It is fun to read and crammed full of thought-provoking, practical and motivating take-aways.
I recommend this book to HR professionals, business leaders, sales leaders, and anyone who is trying to not only navigate the world's economy today, but to succeed in it. With the Six Ps of Progress, Dean gives us all the incredible opportunity to be purposeful in creating progress, not just change, in our lives and work.

If only I had read this book prior to the Tech Bubble burst in 2001. While working at a software company, like many of my fellow HR professionals, I was doing my best to "lead change," to "manage change," in an unprecedented time when high-technology companies dramatically went from such incredible highs on Wall Street to such devastating lows in a short period of time. We were reeling from the emotional shock and uncertainty after the events of 9/11. This book would not only have provided a new way of looking at change management, but also a more hopeful way of beginning to answer the question: "What now?" So here we are again in the midst of unprecedented economic times. HR professionals are again faced with the challenge of managing our workforce in a shrinking economy. *The Progress Challenge* is a must-read for all of us. Only the businesses that are able to grow, gain market share, gain Customer loyalty, and gain Employee loyalty and engagement will survive when recessions occur. That requires more than change management; it requires progress. It requires committing to progress and it requires persistence.

The Progress Challenge

I am so fortunate to be working for Southwest Airlines, a company that truly gets what taking care of Customers and Employees really means in any economy. (For starters, the "C" in Customers and the "E" in Employees are capitalized deliberately.) In describing the 6 P's of Progress (I won't give away too much!), Dean captures why Southwest Airlines Employees provide such incredible Customer Service. We LUV what we do and our Company LUVS us! We work very hard during the selection process to hire Employees with a natural desire to serve others. At Southwest, we hire for attitude and train for skill (as needed). Yeah, some skills are incredibly hard to train, but to train someone to have a great attitude and to enjoy their work, their Customers, and their fellow Employees is completely impossible. The mission of Southwest Airlines is dedication to the highest quality of Customer Service delivered with a sense of warmth, friendliness, individual pride, and Company Spirit. Try doing that with a lousy attitude! Having a Fun-LUVing Attitude is not just part of our "core values," it is a requirement of every Employee.

What Dean explains in a witty and entertaining way is that our attitudes, our ability to endure and successfully emerge from the current recession, our shot at getting what we want out of this life, is up to each one of us. I have always believed that "if it is meant to be, it is up to me." Dean explains why that is true and gives us the tools to make it happen! We have to grab every minute of every day and create progress in our work and in our lives. We own it. I own it. I will be progress. This book is so timely. Thanks, Dean.

-- Julie Weber, Senior Director, People
People & Leadership Development
Southwest Airlines

To Change Is Human; to Progress, Divine.

The Way of
the Donut Man

At about 9:45 a.m. on a cold and super rainy Saturday morning, I got into my car and made the seven-and-a-half-minute trip to my local Blockbuster. I was on a mission to snag, for me and my kids, *Swiss Family Robinson*, an awesome early Disney Classic and a perfect movie for a rainy Saturday.

Blockbuster had not opened yet, so I walked down the sidewalk, checking out the other shops and waiting for 10:00 a.m. when Blockbuster would open. The rain was really coming down, but I stayed dry walking under the shopping center's awning.

About four shops down from Blockbuster, I noticed a small, healthy-looking Korean man who appeared to be about fifty years old. He was standing in front of a little donut shop under the awning. The man was holding a HUGE blue umbrella and facing the rain. The donut shop was the only place open along this strip of shops, and it was packed with people.

Umbrella Man just stood there, full of life, smiling. He was in no hurry; in fact, he seemed to be totally content. As I walked past him, we acknowledged each other and said hello.

My curiosity was piqued.
What was this guy up to?

The Progress Challenge

I looked around. At first I thought maybe he was waiting for one of the other shops to open. But if that was true, *why did he still have the big blue umbrella open?*
Why not just close the big thing and wait?
Plus, his back was to the shops. He was looking out at the parking lot and the rain.

Was he waiting for someone? Maybe, but he seemed really involved in the moment (big smile, eyes wide).

Maybe he liked to watch the rain. (I do.)

Maybe he was waiting for a change in the weather before he headed to his car. *But wasn't that what the big blue umbrella was for?*

Why did he need such a big umbrella, anyway?

Then I remembered a small poster I'd seen on the wall of a call center I did some consulting for:
  We can't promise our customers sunny weather, but we can promise to hold an umbrella over them when it rains.

Suddenly it hit me. I knew what he was up to. I spun around and blurted, *"This is your donut shop!"* (If you know me, you know I blurt.)

The man turned to me, smiled, and said proudly, with a thick Korean accent, *"It is, yes."*

"And you are standing here with the umbrella waiting for your customers."

The Progress Challenge

"*Yes,*" he replied with a real upbeat kick in his voice. "*I go out with my umbrella and bring them in. When they are ready to leave, I walk them to their cars.*"

I paused, nodded, and said, "*Wow. That's really good customer service!*"

He smiled, shook his head, and said, "*No. It is my pleasure.*"

From the look in his eyes and the tone of his voice, I could tell he MEANT it. It was HIS pleasure. He wasn't just holding the umbrella for his customers. He was doing it for himself as well. Serving his customers was serving him. It brought him joy, made him happy. He thrived on it.

Was it good customer service? You bet.
Do you think the customers appreciated it? You bet.
Think it will help inspire loyal customers? You bet.
Will holding that umbrella help make his business more successful? You bet.

All of the above is obviously good for him and his business, but he also found joy in the process. Holding that big umbrella and serving his customers brought him pleasure. He was receiving from his giving. It brought him pleasure to offer and deliver on the promise of pleasure. He was doing good and he knew it. He made "doing good" good for him. The Donut Man wasn't waiting for the weather to change; he was too focused on working and winning.

Offer the Promise of Pleasure.

Meet the Progress Challenge.

The Progress Challenge Revealed

I will get right to the point: The *Progress Challenge* is to **Be Progress**, not merely *make* progress. **BE PROGRESS.** We – along with our ideas, products, and services – must be positioned <u>AS</u> *progress* in the minds of those we wish to inspire to positive action; we must see ourselves as progress in our own minds as well. Our personal progress is directly linked to helping others progress.

This book offers a fresh and powerful blueprint for meeting this *Progress Challenge* while working and winning in this complicated, stress-inducing, world of radical change. Its transferable concepts are offered to help inspire progress-based action within yourself and others, and reap the bounty of higher (and happier) performance levels in your organizations.

There should be some ideas, tips, and strategies in this book that make you think, *"I <u>knew</u> that. That's common sense."* Beware of anything that, after some thought, does NOT seem like common sense. The unfortunate truth about common sense is that it's rarely common practice. The tough journey, in business and in life, is to travel the long road from "always KNEW" to "always DO."

> **"Everybody gets so much information all day long that they lose their common sense."**
> *-- Gertrude Stein*

The Progress Challenge

In these pages, you'll learn how to enhance your opportunities by implementing and using what I call the **Six Ps of Progress**. However, simply learning how to enhance your opportunities by being aware of the Six Ps is not the goal. The goal is to actually enhance your opportunities by using the Six Ps of Progress in your life and work. Execution is vital.

Learning should not lead to simply knowing. Learning should lead to **action.** Working and winning in a world of change requires well-planned, progress-based action.

In a sales call, is the sales professional's main goal for the prospect to know what the sales professional offers? NO! The prospect reaching across the desk, shaking the salesperson's hand and saying, *"Thanks for coming by. Now I KNOW what you do,"* is not why the salesperson shined his shoes or applied her blush. The main goal was for the prospect to:
- Sign up
- Take action
- Buy something
- Request a proposal
- Offer a new contact
- Champion the cause
- Put down a down payment
- Agree to a second meeting
- Move the business relationship forward
- Be inspired to help the relationship progress

It's the same with this book. My aim is for you to USE these concepts to create strong resolve that ignites and sustains progress toward goals, even as the world continues to shift and creak around us.

The Progress Challenge

The Progress Challenge is just that, a challenge – a challenge to progress, a challenge to work and win in this world of continual, mind-spinning change. Meeting this challenge creates better leaders, better team members, better human beings. Being progress for ourselves and others establishes and cements customer loyalty, generates quality referrals, and leads to career development and job satisfaction.

There is a powerful and important connection between solid leadership, sales success, personal motivation, and customer loyalty. All are achieved by effectively positioning ideas, recommendations, solutions, products, services – even ourselves – as progress in the minds of those we wish to inspire to action.

How do we position ourselves, our ideas, our products and services as <u>progress</u>, and not simply as change, in the minds of those we wish to inspire to action?

How can we **Be Progress** *in a world of change?*

Many potent how-to's are offered in this book; however, *The Progress Challenge* is first and foremost a methodology for developing your own personalized how-to's that WORK for you and your team. Use the Six Ps of Progress to help your clients, customers, team members, and coworkers connect with how your ideas and expertise, as well as the action steps you are encouraging them to take, will help them *progress*.

**We work and win when we work to help others win.
We progress as we help others progress.**

Be Progress.

The Progress Challenge

To Change Is Human; to Progress, Divine.

"It is not strange ... to mistake change for progress."
-- *Millard Fillmore*

Change happens. We can't avoid change.

New technologies are created.
Markets bear and bull.
Companies merge.
Organizations come together.
Children are born.
Rain falls. Tides turn. Lives evolve.

We are always in some form of transition, always arriving at some new *place* and dealing with new rollouts, new ideas, new everything. The very molecules inside the cells of our bodies are in constant flux. Our world and our lives are always changing, but they are not always progressing. It is natural to resist what we view as change. However, we embrace what we view as progress.

<u>Progress</u> means: forward movement, advance, gradual betterment. It takes awareness, character, discipline, and effort to progress.

Change is inevitable.
Progress is a choice.

The word *progress* carries a forward thrust and focus, a vibrant and transcendent quality that the words *change* and even *success* don't deliver. With every *success* comes the desire for more success.

The Progress Challenge

When we reach a goal, our natural ambitiousness tells us that the goal is also the stepping stone to the next, possibly more rewarding and worthwhile, goal. Therefore, every success establishes a *new norm,* and brings with it the question: *What next?*

The road to success is always under construction. We are always striving for something. (I will share that the something I am referring to is not a person, place, or thing, but rather a feeling. A mixture of six feelings, to be exact, but we will deal with that soon enough.) Continual striving can become quite unpleasant and unhealthy if we do not take time to soak in the positive buzz – feelings – from our forward momentum.

When we focus on daily progress, we are able to feel daily satisfaction. With every forward step, we see more clearly, our confidence grows, our position improves, and our options multiply. We progress toward today's goal on the strength of our past progress. Once achieved, today's goal becomes tomorrow's launching pad.

> **"Out of every fruition of success, no matter what, comes forth something to make a new effort necessary."**
> *-- Walt Whitman*

When a new opportunity comes our way, we internalize it, and size it up as Progress or Change. This new opportunity could be starting a new relationship, buying an electronic gadget, working extra hours on a project, getting up to speed on a new product line, working to meet quota, anything. **All progress is change, but not all change is progress.**

The Progress Challenge

Let's say I have an upset stomach. *"Man, I've got a stomachache. Ouch! My stomach is killing me. This has got to change."*

Somebody hears me, walks over, and punches me in the nose. *Is that change?* Yeah, it's change. But it's not progress. Well, maybe to the person who punched me, but not to me.

What may seem like progress (good) to one person or group of people may seem like change (bad) to another. Propaganda, book burning, even war and murder are all thought of as "progress" at some point in the minds of the perpetrators (scary). Because progress is subjective, there is no single factor that clearly determines whether an event represents progress or change.
However, we can say that we:
- Start businesses to *progress, not change*
- Hire employees to *progress, not change*
- Work on teams to *progress, not change*
- Make the tough choices and the tough phone calls to *progress, not change*
- Keep our cool when dealing with belligerent customers to *progress, not change*
- Cross the road to *progress, not change*
- Answer the phone to *progress, not change*
- Spend our hard-earned money to *progress, not change*. (<u>We would rather keep our *change* than change, but will offer our best to progress.</u>)
- Diet and exercise to *progress, not change*

As we age we realize that slowing change can be progress. Think of the forty-year-old swimmer who manages to equal her performance from five years before. Maintenance is progress in that it avoids change for the worse.

25

The Progress Challenge

We do not want life-changing products, services, experiences, ideas, and opportunities. We want life-progressing products, services, experiences, ideas and opportunities.

We should be careful not to mistake mere change for progress. Just because something is new or flashy does not mean it is right or adds meaning to our lives. And as my friend and fellow author Shama Hyder says, we do live in a "next big thing" world. However, because all progress is change, people who claim to be 100% "resistant to (any) change" are often choosing to be resistant to the possibility of progress.

To Change Is Human; to Progress, Divine.

Be Progress.

<u>Quick shout out to Alex Pope</u>

If he were among us today, eighteenth-century English poet Alexander Pope would likely be one popular guy on Twitter. It was he who wrote the lofty words, *"To err is human; to forgive, divine."* Pope is said to be the third most frequently quoted writer in the English language, after Shakespeare and Tennyson.

Alexander may not be on Twitter, but I am, follow my blog posts at: Twitter.com/DeanLindsay

Ponder & Progress: Progress or Change?

1. What transitions are most significant in the world?

2. What transitions do you see in your professional life?

3. What transitions are shaping your personal life?

4. How can you focus on daily progress?

5. What "next big thing" means progress for you?

6. What "next big thing" would <u>not</u> be progress for you?

7. What are you striving for?

8. What's next? Why?

9. What does progress mean to you?

10. Which parts of your life are progressing and which are merely changing?

"We all want progress, but if you're on the wrong road, progress means doing an about-turn and walking back to the right road; in that case, the man who turns back soonest is the most progressive."
-- C.S. Lewis

The Progress Challenge

Reasons Create Movement
Motivated to Progress?

I read a funny cartoon in *Fast Company* magazine a good while back. It was of two fish swimming next to each other. One of the fish had a hook dangling from its mouth. That fish said, *"Oh, it was a scary couple of minutes, but now I am making a fortune as a motivational speaker."*

Several times over the years I have been referred to as a *Motivational Speaker* and at first I really didn't care for it. I had this image of a *Motivational Speaker* as being a kind of smarmy, slightly plastic and over-the-top *"people person,"* who sprinted through crowds giving everybody high fives, before ascending to the podium to share his rags-to-riches-to-rags-to-riches story. He or she might then encourage seminar goers to turn to their neighbor and repeat a soulful mantra like, *"I am. I will. I can,"* followed by a cleansing breath, a mindful hokey pokey, the sharing of a deep secret and a good cathartic cry.

But as I sought the fundamental meaning of being motivational, I came to realize that each of us has the need and the opportunity to be motivational every day of our lives.
- Good leaders are motivational
- Good parents are motivational
- Good sales professionals are motivational
- Good customer-service representatives are motivational
- Good teachers are motivational

I sure as heck better be motivational. You better be, too. *Why else would others listen to us, utilize our services, hire us, be led by us?*

The Progress Challenge

We each may be motivational, but the decision to be motivated is a personal choice. I can't motivate you and you can't motivate me. I may be motivational. You may be motivational. But truly, no one IS a motivator. The only person who can actually motivate you is you.

> "Motivation is a fire from within. If someone else tries to light that fire under you, chances are it will burn very briefly."
> -- *Stephen Covey*

The word motivation can be broken down into two root words: Motive and Action.

Motive is an inner drive that prompts a person to *act* in a certain way. Motive is the goal or object of one's action. Other words for motive include reasons, purpose, intention.

Action is simply the doing of something. *Examples of actions include:* Do, rent, read, act, try, sign up, show up, eat, move.

Motivation, therefore, is the *inner drive to act, to do, to try.*

Simply put:
Reasons create movement.

As William Shakespeare wrote in *The Life and Death of King John,* "*Strong reasons make strong actions.*" Often we fixate on a goal without giving enough focus and attention to the reasons behind the goal.

It is not a goal that motivates us, but our internalized reasons behind the goal that propel us to action.

The Progress Challenge

As we connect with the fact that our internal reasons inspire our external actions, we begin to notice that our true enemies come from within. Among these resident vixens:
- Self-doubt
- Fear & Anxiety
- Impatience
- Lack of focus
- Procrastination
- Stress
- Poor self-management (time management)
- Misguided pursuit of perfection
- Fear of success

Many of us do not need to come to terms with the world around us. Instead, we need to come to terms with our own unrealistic expectations and poorly defined goals. Well-established reasons help us feel the internal pressure needed to focus.

We must dig to the roots and remind ourselves of the benefits, the reasons behind the actions that will move us forward. We need to do this for those we wish to inspire to action also. Being able to share with customers, clients, coworkers, and employees how they will be able to move forward by partnering with us is a major key to working and winning in this challenging world of change.

There is always some movement, but it is not always forward. Strengthen your commitment by continually reminding yourself of the personal benefits that reaching your and/or your company's goals will have in your life. Each day we have the choice to move forward.

Be Progress.

Ponder & Progress: Reasons Create Movement

1. What are your reasons behind your goals?

2. How are your reasons propelling you to action?

3. How can you become more motivated and bound to your goals?

4. How can you help others discover, realize, and embrace their own reasons for action?

5. What is your WHY?

6. What are the reasons behind your movement?

7. What strong reasons do you need to take strong actions?

8. How do you create inner drive?

9. How are you encouraging others to develop inner drive?

10. What are you motivated to do? Why?

"He who has a why to live for can bear almost any how."
-- Frederick Nietzsche

Becoming a Progress Agent

The people we desire to inspire to action (lead, do business with, etc.) must believe that our ideas, our products, our services, our leadership, and our initiatives will help them to move forward. Solid trust must be in place before we can even hope others will choose to alter their lives to include us.

**We must be seen as catalysts in others' progress, agents in their progress.
We must be _Progress Agents._**

Progress Agents practice a "live and help progress" philosophy. We thrive on being able to take a challenging situation and proactively work to create outcomes that are positive for all involved (including ourselves). We consistently say and do the things that we believe will help our companies, as well as clients and coworkers, to grow, advance, make headway, become better, make strides, and progress in this world of change.

Progress Agents understand that trust is the basis for all positive long-term relationships (even the one we have with ourselves). We know that the key to meeting the progress challenge is to have others _trust_ that we ARE and will continue to _Be Progress_. Progress Agents know that trust is the **_promise of progress_**, but not a guarantee of progress. Trust is fragile, but is strengthened by continually being progress for ourselves and others.

The Progress Challenge

Progress Agents learn about customers, prospects, employees, coworkers, and even friends, uncovering their unique ***parameters for progress.*** The more we can get into the shoes, hearts, and heads of the people we wish to inspire to action, the more we can know what progress means <u>to them.</u> We are then able to relate in ways that show how our initiatives, ideas, products, and services are beneficial and valuable to them.

Ponder & Progress:
Uncovering Others' Parameters for Progress

1. *What does progress mean to the people you wish to inspire to action?*

2. *What are they going for in life?*

3. *What are their interests?*

4. *What are their goals?*

5. *What are they striving for?*

6. *What are their reasons for movement?*

7. *How are their reasons propelling them into action?*

8. *How can you share how your products and services are progress for the people you wish to inspire to action?*

9. *How can you share how your ideas, recommendations, and solutions are progress?*

10. *How can you become a Progress Agent in their minds?*

The Rise of Progress Leadership
Change Management Is Dead

The business term *change management* has been around for a good long while. The term relates to *"initiating significant change"* within an organization's processes. This change can include anything from altering work culture to embracing diversity to modifying an individual's work tasks to increasing company morale and loyalty. The goal of *"initiating significant change"* is solid, but where is the passion in the word choice?

The problem with the term "change management" is that no one really desires to change or plans to change. We desire and plan to *progress*.

**We do not want managers to manage our change.
We want leaders to lead our progress.**

Let's call *"initiating significant change"* what it truly is (or should be): **Progress Leadership.** In a time of continual transformation, committed leaders – Progress Agents – should focus on inspiring the progress, not apologizing for the change. Progress Agents don't just TELL people what to do. Progress Agents include others in the *progress* as well as the *process*. It is <u>reasons</u> that shape, nourish, and sustain the thoughts that create the actions necessary to reach desired results.

> "If you want to build a ship, don't drum up people together to collect wood and don't assign them tasks and work, but rather teach them to long for the endless immensity of the sea."
> -- *Antoine de Saint-Exupéry*

The Progress Challenge – Progress Leadership

Companies are most successful at *"initiating significant change"* when the <u>reasons to act</u> connect personally with the individual employees making the alteration in behavior. If the reasons don't connect with the individual, then the *planned progress* will be viewed as merely change and will be resisted or at least not acted on. Team members may still physically clock in but have often mentally checked out.

Progress Agents work to positively influence thoughts and feelings as well as oversee actions. We live in a world of influence. We are influenced to purchase this, to believe that, to participate in this activity, to attend that event. This is not a bad thing. Most often it is good. Our parents influenced our decision not to play with fire. Our best friend influenced our decision not to wear corduroy. *Ever turned a friend on to a restaurant?* You influenced your friend. *Ever go to a movie because a friend said it was good?* That friend influenced you.

"There is only one way... to get anybody to do anything. And that is by making the other person want to do it."
-- *Dale Carnegie*

Dale Carnegie wrote his classic *How to Win Friends and Influence People* way back in 1936, and its wisdom is no less true and vibrantly powerful today. The book is packed with insight on leading and building strong relationships by lifting people up, making them feel good, and "spurring people on to success." Wisely, the book is not called *How to Lift People Up and Make Them Feel Good* or *How to Spur People on to Success.* No, Carnegie's classic is appropriately titled: *How to <u>Win</u> Friends and <u>Influence</u> People. And who is doing the winning?* It's you and me, along with the person being lifted up, made to feel good, and spurred on to success (*read: influenced and led*).

The Progress Challenge – Progress Leadership

In his book, Mr. Carnegie encourages us to, among other things: *Talk in terms of the other person's interests, respect others' opinions, try honestly to see things from the other person's point of view, and try to make the other person happy about doing the things you suggest.* In other words, genuinely care about people and their feelings.

But Mr. Carnegie's classic does not only encourage us to take these actions for the benefit of the people we are respecting and "making happy." The book doesn't even make the argument that it is even morally right to care about people's feelings *(although I am sure Mr. Carnegie would agree that it is)*. No, the book simply makes the clear case that caring about others' feelings is good for the person (or company) who cares.

Intense focus on feelings in a time of transformation is often described as the *"human side of change management."* This always gives me pause.

The "human side" of business—what other side is there? Some might say the company side.

So then, the company and the humans are on different sides? That's the problem right there. Companies are formed by people (humans) partnering to get their wants and needs met by helping other people (humans) get their wants and needs met. Leaders who do not take the individual into account and do not plan for the human side of *Progress* often find themselves scratching their heads about where their plans went wrong.

> **"Humanize globalization and globalize humanization."**
> -- Father Anselm Gruen

The Progress Challenge – Progress Leadership

It takes more than the title of supervisor, manager, or "change agent" to lead people in the direction of progress. We all want to be in relationships with people, as well as partner with organizations that bring progress to our lives.

Without personal commitment to execute, new organizational plans and initiatives often fail. Execution is assured by establishing clear links between operations, strategy, and team members. Progress leadership means working to understand and communicate how a team member's personal goals can dovetail with the organization's goals and thus create true commitment that gets the team member to act – because he or she wants to, not because they have to. Progress Leadership means striving to help others find meaning in their work.

> "Meaning arises when people bring together what they do with what is important to them."
> *-- Viktor Frankl*
> *(More on the illuminating work and life of Dr. Frankl on pages 48-49 and 107-112)*

Also, just because a company is getting bigger does not mean it is progressing. A serious challenge for companies large and small is to progress, and not just change. Moving our focus from change management to progress leadership creates a shift in power from wielding power over employees to creating power among employees. Progress Agents thus create a work culture in which empowered employees are committed to finding what is truly the next step forward.

Goodbye, Change Management. Hello, Progress Leadership!

Super Quick Action Steps to Excelling at Progress Leadership

Focus on Inspiring Progress
(rather than apologizing for change).

Care and Listen. Care and Listen Some More.

Get to Know Team Members' Parameters for Progress.

Help Establish Team Member Expectations.

Internalize, but Do Not Personalize.
(Work to not take stuff too personally, even when someone means it personally.)

Drink Water. Drink More Water.

Be Passionate About Your Work.

Be Passionate About Your Team.

Be Passionate About Your LIFE.

Compliment with Reason.

Smile with Reason.

Get Enough Sleep.

Read Good Stuff.

Be Patient.

The Progress Challenge – Progress Leadership

Exercise.

Feel Sharp.

Look Sharp.

Be a Progress Agent.

Share Your Expertise.

Accentuate the Progress.

Be Human. Be Humane.

Eat Right. Eat Breakfast.

Maximize Your Personal Potential.

Get a Massage. Get Another Massage.

Ask Questions that Show Respect and Value.

Surround Yourself with Self-Motivating Experts.

Cherish and Cultivate Constructive Communication.

Craft Progress-Based Personal & Organizational Goals.

Help Others Choose to Feel Positive About
Their Work and Lives.

Meet the Progress Challenge.

Be Progress.

Partnering to Progress

> "Give me a stock clerk with a goal and I'll give you a man who will make history. Give me a man with no goals and I'll give you a stock clerk."
> -- J.C. Penney

Each of us has personal goals. The company we partner with (work for) has organizational goals. This is not a problem. This should be great news. One of the most effective ways to progress toward our personal goals is by <u>partnering</u> with our organizations. You might say, *"Hold on, Deano. I work there, but I don't partner with them."* Not true.

We *work* there because we believe that by accomplishing team goals, we take steps closer to our personal goals. If we didn't believe that way, we wouldn't (or at least shouldn't) work there. True, the relationship between employee and employer is sometimes one of conflict, with a worker doing a particular job because they need the money and don't think they can get anything better elsewhere. But at every level, everyone *works* to personally progress. Even the CEO is there because she believes that by partnering with the company, she takes solid steps toward her own personal goals.

Organizations are only as strong as their team members' personal goals and the team members' belief that the organization's progress helps them progress toward those goals.

The Progress Challenge – Partnering to Progress

People without personal goals are "no show" employees, poor salespeople, and inconsistent customer-service professionals. That's a major reason that teenagers *sometimes* don't make the best employees. It's not because they are lazy (though some are, as are some adults) or do not have any work ethic. It's because they generally don't have strong reasons connected to the work they do. On the other hand, let's say that a 15-year-old boy wants a car on his 16th birthday and he has to buy it himself. He is *committed* to getting that car.

Will he be a reliable employee? Likely, yes.

Why? Because he is committed and connected to the outcome of the work. He is partnering to progress.

For teams to progress, team members must believe that they are personally progressing. Team members must believe that as they strive to accomplish team goals, they are taking steps toward their own personal goals. If a company's goals don't line up with its team members' personal goals (and vice versa), neither is likely to be reached.

Sales managers should love it when their sales professionals: buy a new house, have their eye on a boat, or decide to have another kid, because now that person has some strong reasons to take strong action. They have strong *whys* to get out there and sell.

When our company has a new product rollout, is merging with another company, or has a new way to get business moving, it is natural to think, *Oh, no! Here comes something else I have to learn. Something else I have to do.*

The Progress Challenge – Partnering to Progress

But think about it. Wouldn't it be far worse if the leadership within our companies said, *"We have no new ideas on how to be profitable. We have no new ideas on how to progress. Go get 'em, tiger!"*?

We should be glad, excited, and even relieved about new initiatives, because the decision makers *(who should know a thing or three)* believe they have ideas that will help the company progress, and in turn help us to progress.

Without our "work," we would still have our personal goals. Even if we were "trust-fund kids," we would have to find some other way to take progressive steps.

We partner with our organizations because we have goals, and through our partnering we take steps to achieving them. Companies with solid, well-thought-out organizational goals make it easier for us to achieve our goals. The company helps us progress as we help the company progress.

Partner and Progress.

The Progress Challenge – Partnering to Progress

Ponder & Progress: Partnering to Progress

1. Why do you "work?"

2. How are you <u>progress</u> for your organization?

3. How is your organization <u>progress</u> for you?

4. How are you <u>progress</u> for those you "work" with?

5. What are two of your organization's goals?

6. How can working toward these organizational goals become steps toward your personal goals?

7. How will accomplishing these organizational goals accelerate the achievement of your personal goals?

8. Does your organization help you avoid pain? How?

9. What organizational initiatives have you resisted that could lead to your personal progress?

10. How are you a Progress Agent at work?

"You have to accept that no matter where you work, you are not an employee; you are in a business with one employee – yourself."
-- *Andrew S. Grove*

The Six Ps of Progress

The Progress Principle
Introducing the Six Ps of Progress

The Progress Principle: Everything we do is done because we believe, consciously, or more often subconsciously, that the *projected consequences* of those actions will be us feeling the *right* mixture of six core feelings, feelings I call:

The **Six Ps of Progress** ™
    Peace of Mind
    Pleasure
    Profit
    Prestige
    Pain Avoidance
    Power

We project consequences based on past experiences, education, the influence of others, and our imagination. *Projected consequences* are the results we think will occur. We project consequences, we take the action, and then we perceive the actual consequences. The actual consequences may not be what we'd expected the consequences would be, but there are *always* consequences, and some blend of the *Six Ps of Progress* is experienced.

What makes *The Progress Principle* a challenge is that feeling the right blend of the *Six Ps of Progress* is often not achieved when the feeling of them is the goal. The right blend is more often felt as a by-product of working toward and attaining a goal. This is why we are compelled to:
- Strive for Significance
- Pursue a Higher Purpose
- Craft and Commit to Goals
- Work to Progress.

The Six Ps of Progress

I arrived at *The Progress Principle* as well as the *Six Ps of Progress* after spending years aggressively researching the works of many of the world's top minds on the subjects of motivation and commitment. In my studies I found myself leaning heavily on the work of Austrian psychiatrist and neurologist Viktor Frankl, the founder of Logotherapy.

> **"For the meaning of life differs from man to man, from day to day and from hour to hour. What matters, therefore, is not the meaning of life in general but rather the specific meaning of a person's life at a given moment."**
> -- *Viktor Frankl*

I believe it is through our desire to feel the *Six Ps of Progress*, mixed with our belief in how to feel them, that we establish what Viktor Frankl calls our "meaning" at any given moment. I devote several pages to this amazing man's views, life, and work later in this book (page 107 for you book-skipper-arounders).

Though much of my study of Frankl's work has been self study, I had the privilege of participating in both the Thirteenth and Seventeenth World Congresses on Viktor Frankl's Logotherapy. It was at the Thirteenth World Congress that I first met the president of the International Board of Directors of the Viktor Frankl Institute of Logotherapy, Robert Barnes, Ph.D., and his wife, Dorothy Barnes, Ed.D. (who also serves on the Institute's International Board).

I was the only one at the World Congress with no letters (Ph.D., Ed.D., etc.) attached to their name. *(Well, I am Jerry Dean Lindsay, Jr., but that wasn't helpful in that group.)*

The Six Ps of Progress

The Barneses quickly befriended me and even invited me to lunch with them. Over our lunch, they showed great interest in how I came to know so much about Frankl's work and why I was attending the Congress. I told them of my studies and sheepishly shared with these two revered educators The Progress Principle, my concept of the *Six Ps of Progress*. I also explained how I believed our desire to feel these feelings helps us establish meaning, which propels us to action. Robert smiled widely, nodded, and seemed pleased. Dorothy smiled as well, but also seemed to be mulling over the Six Ps in her brain.

Our conversation went in a couple of different directions for a while – family, travel – and then Dorothy said quite confidently, *"Dean, I believe you are on to something with your Six Ps of Progress and here's why. For several years, I had wanted to lose a few pounds. However, it wasn't until Robert and I began to discuss the need to have a 30th wedding anniversary portrait taken that I actually took action. The reason I finally took action was that I knew the picture would get printed in the paper because it was our 30th, and I knew the whole community, as well as all our friends, would see it. I wanted the pleasure and prestige connected with looking good in that photo. I also wanted to avoid the pain of not looking good to myself in that photo. Good work, Dean."* Dr. Robert Barnes smiled again, nodded, and seemed pleased.

I, on the other hand, was stunned. *"Wow, thank you!"* I was thrilled. It was the first time someone that I was certain KNEW what they were talking about told me they thought I was on to something. I have often thought about that lunch and conversation with great gratitude. *Thank you, Dr. and Dr. Barnes.*

The Six Ps of Progress

Marketing and advertising professionals know about the *Six Ps of Progress* (*though they don't call them that...yet*). Every good commercial comes down to showing how a particular product or service can help the buyer progress toward feeling pleasure, peace of mind, profit, prestige, and power, while also limiting or avoiding pain. We choose from an endless list of possible actions in order to try and achieve our desired outcomes, thereby feeling the *Six Ps of Progress*. Some of these actions might include:

- *Volunteering at a food bank*
- *Dealing with an upset customer*
- *Cleaning out the garage*
- *Making sales calls*
- *Eating out*
- *Reading to our kids*
- *Praying*
- *Paying our taxes*
- *Feeding the pig*
- *Sleeping*
- *Watching a movie*
- *Signing a contract*
- *Lifting weights*
- *Going Green*
- *Writing this book*
- *Hanging out on Facebook*
- *Doing laundry*
- *Hiring a new employee*
- *Firing an employee*
- *Buying a new pair of shoes*
- *Picking up trash*
- *WHATEVER*

Each of these actions has positive meaning only when we believe it will help us feel a mixture of the Six Ps of Progress.

The Six Ps of Progress

We are all motivated by self-interest. This does not have to be selfish thinking. Even if our desired outcome is for someone else to feel pleasure or avoid pain, this too is connected to us feeling an empathetic mixture of pleasure, peace of mind, profit, prestige, power, and pain avoidance. If it weren't, we wouldn't act. **We give not so much out of the goodness of our hearts as for the goodness we feel in our hearts when we give.**

Most of us know that giving adds great pleasure to life and that a life of serving others also offers great profit and even helps avoid pain. In fact, as we begin to understand this, we see how the biggest givers end up with the most.

> **"You can get everything in life you want, if you help enough other people get what they want."**
> -- Zig Ziglar
> *(I know this quote is over-quoted, but it goes perfectly here, and Zig is right on the mark.)*

A major hurdle to *being progress* for ourselves and others is that nothing actually <u>causes</u> someone to feel the *Six Ps of Progress*. Products, services, ideas, and companies can *offer* pleasure, peace of mind, profit, prestige, pain avoidance, and power. But they do not inherently *cause* it, just like nothing exterior actually *causes* stress or happiness.

What brings peace or prestige to you might not do it for me. For example: *How much money will make you feel "in the money," or feel peace of mind?* Various studies have determined that no matter what their annual income, the majority of people say they'd be significantly happier and more content if they only had *one-third more* in salary, in their nest egg, tucked under the mattress, etc.

The Six Ps of Progress

The fact is, feeling the Six Ps is entirely *our* choice, and with the power of choice comes the challenge to progress. It is in the ways we go about meeting this Progress Challenge that we establish an action's meaning, and even the meaning of our life. Each of us makes decisions as to what to wear, whom to connect with, what to invest our time in, whom to help, and whom not to help based on whether we believe, consciously or subconsciously, that these acts will bring us these *Six Ps of Progress* – short-term or long-term.

At a mostly subconscious level, we are continuously thinking to ourselves: *Does taking this action (buying this product, switching vendors, hiring this person, calling this help line, agreeing to these terms, etc.) help me move toward pleasure, peace of mind, profit, prestige, and power, or help me to avoid pain?*

And in so doing, we are basically asking ourselves:
**Will taking this action lead to Progress,
or will it merely lead to more change?**

<u>Note on Progress:</u>
Along with the work of Viktor Frankl, I avidly studied the thoughts of Tom Peters, Leo Buscaglia, Tony Robbins, W. Edwards Deming, Tom Hopkins, John Maxwell, Wayne Dyer, Og Mandino, Ken Blanchard, Denis Waitley, and the one and only Mr. Zig Ziglar. In an attempt to soak in their concepts subconsciously while I slept, I would even go to sleep with one of these superstars waxing poetic on my tape player (yes, tapes – this was a while ago). I don't know if it helped. I do know it didn't hurt, though it was a little odd to wake up to Leo Buscaglia shouting that he loved me. (He loved you, too. Leo loved everyone!)

Let's take a closer look at the Six Ps of Progress.

Peace of Mind

> "Every goal, every action, every thought, every feeling one experiences, whether it be consciously or unconsciously known, is an attempt to increase one's level of peace of mind."
> -- *Sidney Madwed*

If I had to choose one of the *Six Ps of Progress* that was the most often strived for, it would be Peace of Mind. In simple terms, *peace of mind* is acceptance and contentment. Peace of mind means inner calmness, quiet mind, serenity, a clear conscience, safety, composure, contentment. It also means an absence of mental stress or anxiety, a lack of agitation. (Sounds nice, huh?)

Peace of mind is the state of tranquility and harmony, sleeping easy at night, living easy during the day. When I think of an example of someone who seems to enjoy peace of mind, I think of Jimmy Buffett. I am sure Jimmy has had a bad day here and there, even in Margaritaville, but I have a hard time imagining him not eventually finding that lost shaker of salt – or at least taking its loss with a grain of salt.

Strong relationships offer peace of mind. Insurance offers peace of mind. Good benefit packages offer peace of mind. Money in the bank offers peace of mind. Good buzz in our industries offers peace of mind. Meaningful work offers peace of mind. Seatbelts offer peace of mind. Receiving top-notch prequalified quality referrals offers peace of mind. Receiving solid customer service offers peace of mind. In equal measure, I strongly believe that *delivering* solid customer service offers peace of mind.

The Six Ps of Progress – Peace of Mind

Most would agree that having peace of mind is healthy and the opposite of being anxious or burdened with regret and worry. Understanding that unexpected things will happen, markets shift, wells dry up – and that all we truly control is our actions and reactions – offers peace of mind. We have the best shot at feeling peace of mind when we start viewing the world and its opportunities from a healthy and useful perspective.

> **"For peace of mind, resign as general manager of the universe."**
> *--Larry Eisenberg*

Peace of mind may also relate to a state of being spiritual, or having a sense of possessing enough knowledge and understanding to keep oneself positive and centered in the face of stressful stimuli and discord. It is tough to feel peace when we are angry or upset. Forgiving both ourselves and others, as well as letting go of grudges, are prerequisites to peace of mind.

Peace of mind does not suggest lack of awareness, Pollyannaism, or loss of touch with reality. Someone with peace of mind can be extremely aware and closely connected to the reality of the times. Belief in ourselves and our abilities to make good choices despite any downturn or misstep offers peace of mind. Knowing we are doing our best at becoming our best selves is, in itself, peace of mind. Believing we can work and win in a world of change sustains our peace with courage and conviction.

Offer the Promise of Peace of Mind.

Be Progress.

The Six Ps of Progress – Peace of Mind

The Way of Customer Care
Earning and Maintaining Customer Loyalty

Peace of mind is as oxygen in the challenging world of customer service. Sure, pleasure, profit, prestige, pain avoidance, and power are desired too, but first and foremost, customers need the peace and confidence that only our caring can provide. Continually showing them that we care, are knowledgeable, and are committed to their progress is the vital force that keeps our relationships and businesses alive. And I know what I'm talking about. I do not wish to brag, but I am a customer. I have been since I got my first allowance. *Heck, a couple of you may be customers too.*

As customers, we want the peace of mind that comes from a customer-service representative listening to our issues and championing our cause. We want the peace of mind that comes from believing that a sales representative is acting in our best interest. We want the peace of mind that comes from employees looking and acting like they want to be there, and who are passionate about their work.

But let's not think for a minute that providing solid customer service is something done *only* for the customer. We shouldn't kid ourselves. Providing solid customer care adds to our peace of mind, too. Many of our goals are achieved by serving customers. One of the major reasons we even wear the *"Serve others"* hat is so that later in the day we can wear the *"Serve me"* hat. Our service to others, serves us. It helps to keep the personal benefits of providing unparalleled service front and center in our minds.

The Six Ps of Progress – Peace of Mind

There are times we do not feel like serving customers, but we always want to serve ourselves. There are even times when the customer (who may be surly, rude, drunk) does not deserve our best. But we always desire the best for ourselves. Therefore, it can be helpful to remind ourselves of the role that earning and maintaining customer loyalty plays in our personal peace of mind and progress.

Want to get closer to job security? Serve customers.
Want less stress? Provide commendable customer service.
Want your 401(K) to grow? Serve, earn customer loyalty.
Worried about downsizing? Serve customers.
Want your company to be more profitable? Ditto.
How about better tips? Same.
Want to have more fun at work? Serve those bosses, I mean customers, I mean bosses.
Want more money for advertising? Help, serve, and be progress for customers.
Want to diminish the need for advertising? Be progress.
Want job satisfaction? Serve.
Want your customers to feel peace of mind? Serve.
Do you want the peace of mind that comes with customer loyalty? You guessed it…**Serve Those Customers!**

"There is only one boss – the customer. And he can fire everybody in the company – from the chairman on down – simply by spending his money somewhere else."
-- Sam Walton

Offering customers the promise of peace of mind, offers us peace of mind. That is why we strive for customer loyalty, so that we KNOW we have a customer base that is solid, jazzed, and growing. That knowledge sure helps me sleep well at night. *How about you?*

The Six Ps of Progress – Peace of Mind

Customer service pays off – and not only in spades. In the hand that we deal are the "hearts" of much happier customers and a more satisfying workday; the "diamonds" of higher pay and lower turnover; and the "lucky" clover (club) of more sales and company growth. *(That was forced, but fun.)*

When we lose sight of the personal motivation involved in this game *(ok, I'll stop)* of quality service, we begin to disregard the concerns of our customers. Unfortunately for everyone, this makes them unhappy, leads to legitimate complaints, and could easily end in our looking for some other line of work.

Customer service is far too often a sticky slow web of surly, under-informed customer-service reps, reading in a monotone from a script. Add to that the annoying on-hold music, outdated computer programs, and hard-to-navigate Web sites (none of which offer customers peace of mind or any of the other Six Ps), and you have the perfect Rx for customer *disservice,* also known as failure. Customers with concerns are left feeling stressed and helpless, and with the belief that companies truly don't give a hoot about their well-being.

Just saying we provide good customer service doesn't cut it anymore. Every company, every organization says they provide good customer service, or *great* customer service, or even *stellar* customer service.

You never hear of a company touting their lame service. *"Our customer service generally sucks. But we do have our good days, so how's about buying something?"*

The Six Ps of Progress – Peace of Mind

Many adjectives have been plopped in front of the words "customer service" to help rally some form of interest in providing positive service to customers. They include: Astonishing, Superior, Exceptional, Positively Outrageous, Super, Multicultural, World-Class, Magnetic, Effective, Branded, Practical, Nonpareil, Breakthrough, Remarkable, Magical, Quality, Effective, Five-Star, and Not So Cruddy.

(OK. I made up that last one, but you just wait. Someone will snag it. Next year you'll see an ad for a hot new business book: *Not So Cruddy Service: 7 Habits of Barely Tolerable Service Professionals*.)

A thorough definition of *customer service* is full of intangibles, and it is those intangibles that make or break a business. In today's competitive marketplace, *service* is the most important thing a company has to *offer*.

**Progress in service leads
to progress in sales.**

Many companies win customers with special offers, only to lose that new business to their competitor by providing lousy service. Quality customer service makes the all-important difference when two, ten, or twenty businesses seem to offer the same product or professional service.

The need is undeniable, the concepts are easy to understand, and the training sound, but still, proactive customer service is just not happening. All expect good service but few are willing to give it. It helps to widen our perspective as to what a customer is.

The Six Ps of Progress – Peace of Mind

Anyone affected, positively or negatively, by the work we do (including our families and ourselves) can be thought of as our "customer." Within this wider perspective, we see that real service is based on integrity, care, and sincerity, none of which can be measured with money. Nor can it be automated, no matter how soft-spoken and attractive the audio-animatronic voice may be.

Unfortunately, it seems that when an organization labels some of its professionals as *customer-service reps* or *customer advocates,* the rest of the organization assumes they are let off of the "customer care" hook. Not true. We are ALL in the customer-service business. There is no other business. In fact, there is NO business without the customer.

Every member of our organization is a "customer-service representative," no matter what their title or job description may be. We are all working for the man (or woman), and that person's name is customer *(or client, or guest, or partner, or stockholder, or employee, or team member).*

Customers are not dependent on us; we are dependent on them. But don't get me wrong! An attitude of service is not one of servitude. It is an attitude of goodwill and good-willingness, a willingness to help others progress.

Earn and Maintain Customer Loyalty.

Offer the Promise of Peace of Mind.

Be Progress.

The Six Ps of Progress – Peace of Mind

<u>Ponder & Progress:
Defining Your Way of Customer Care</u>

1. Why do you serve?

2. Whom do you serve?

3. Who are your customers? Who are not your customers?

4. Who should provide customer service?

5. How would you define customer service as a customer?

6. How would you define service as a business owner, customer-service representative or sales professional?

7. Who at your company does not need to be focused on customer service?

8. What are the personal and/or shared rewards of serving customers successfully?

9. What are the consequences of failing to provide what the customer views as "good service?"

10. How is providing solid customer service <u>progress</u> for YOU?

> "The customers are the most important part of the production line."
> -- W. Edwards Deming

The Six Ps of Progress – Peace of Mind

As a service to whomever decides to write
Not So Cruddy Service:
7 Habits of Barely Tolerable Service Professionals,
here is an outline of the 7 Habits.

<u>Habit 1:</u>
Be Slow to React to Customer Concerns

<u>Habit 2:</u>
Begin with the End of the Business Day in Mind

<u>Habit 3:</u>
Put First Things Last and Don't Get Around to Them

<u>Habit 4:</u>
Think Lose/Win or Win/Lose – Somebody Has Got to Lose

<u>Habit 5:</u>
Seek First to Tell. Then Hang Up

<u>Habit 6:</u>
Scrutinize Customer Needs to See If They Warrant Effort

<u>Habit 7:</u>
Sharpen the Tongue to Use on Customers and Coworkers

Ponder & Progress: The Peace of Mind 10

1. How do you, your services, your ideas, your products, your leadership style, your business plan and culture offer others peace of mind?

2. Is there peace of mind to be gained from working with you and for you? Oh, yeah? Like what?

3. How can you and your organization be better positioned as Agents of Peace of Mind in the minds of those you wish to inspire to action?

4. Do customers, clients, and guests take comfort or feel at ease knowing that you and your company are on the case? How so?

5. How is accomplishing the goals you are committed to going to bring you peace of mind?

6. How is working toward your goals bringing you peace of mind?

7. How can you help coworkers, employees, and customers feel more peace of mind in their work – and in their working relationship with you?

8. What aspect of your life and business should you improve to gain more peace of mind?

9. How is your customer service (internal and external) a catalyst for others to feel peace of mind?

10. How do you offer the Promise of Peace of Mind?

The Six Ps of Progress – Pleasure

Pleasure

Humor, good hygiene, clean stores (inside and out), solid eye contact, fair pricing, friendly polite coworkers and customer-service representatives, and leaders who truly care about the well-being of the people they lead, all act to encourage others to feel pleasure. Pleasure is a state of gratification, delight, joy, gladness, satisfaction. Pleasure can come in mental, physical, sensual, or emotional experiences. Pleasure can come from worldly or frivolous delights, recreation, amusement, even diversions.
There can be pleasure in achievement and in having done something "good."

A challenge to offering pleasure is that it is derived from *one's own* liking, as are all the *Six Ps of Progress*. Pleasure can be promoted in countless ways, depending on how a person senses the feeling of pleasure. Some individuals feel pleasure through personal recognition, comfort, entertainment, games, hobbies, accomplishment, and service. Music, sex, taking drugs, writing, jogging, eating Twinkies®, and practically every other imaginable activity, even forms of pain, can bring about the feeling of pleasure. By getting to know those we wish to inspire to action, we are able to share, in ways that are that healthy for them, how we offer them pleasure.

The Promise of Pleasure is why we – and especially customer-service reps – are encouraged to "smile into the phone." When we smile into the phone, there is a little lilt in our voice. The person on the other end of the call can hear that little lilt. That little lilt offers pleasure.

The Six Ps of Progress – Pleasure

Offering the promise of pleasure is profitable. A dissatisfied (sometimes referred to as complaining) customer will explain their point in a more civil way if the person receiving the feedback is pleasurable to talk to. The opposite of pleasure is displeasure. Less-qualified competitors gain our customers purely because someone on our side was offering poor customer service, which caused the customer to feel displeasure.

There can and should be pleasure in service. Find pleasure in pleasing. Savor the opportunity to help coworkers and employees, as well as customers, to progress. We can choose to feel pleasure from the work we do as well as the people we do it with. When traveling internationally on business, I am frequently asked, when getting my passport stamped, if I am traveling for *business or pleasure*. I am always tempted to say *Both*. I like the work I do. It brings me a great deal of pleasure. I hope yours does too.

It is much easier to be working and winning when we are working and grinning.

Joy is a wonderful motivator. Most of us participate best in a positive, upbeat working environment where we feel we are being heard and appreciated. *So why not create some hoopla, have some laughs?* Find the relish in your work. Be the cause of enjoyment. *Where is the whoopee?*

Southwest Airlines is often cited as having an upbeat and caring culture. *Do you know who benefits the most from the Southwest Airlines culture?* Not us, though we get good pricing, friendly customer service, and on-time flights.

The Six Ps of Progress – Pleasure

The group that benefits *most* from the Southwest culture is the Southwest Airlines team members. They all *(well most, anyway)* really get a kick out of their jobs. They gain a great deal of pleasure (as well as the other *Ps of Progress*) from being a Southwest team member.

Southwest believes, *and rightfully so,* that if a company truly takes care of its employees, the employees will take care of the customers. (By the way, this is good for stockholders, too.)

> **"Work is either fun or drudgery. It depends on your attitude. I like fun."**
> *-- Colleen Barrett*
> *(Southwest Airlines' former president, and with the airline since its 1971 inception)*

Plus, the word is out on the street. When a Southwest employee shares where he or she works, people say, *"You work at Southwest? Cool. Great company. Seems like a fun place to work. You guys are well taken care of. You must dig it."* That not only delivers pleasure, but also prestige.

The exact opposite happens when an employee of more than a couple of other airlines shares the same info. It is usually followed by a sympathetic silence, and responses like, *"You guys got problems. You need to work on your customer service. Your executives are abusing you. Are you looking for a new job?"* Bummer.

No fun. No pleasure, no prestige, little promise of progress. Little incentive to strive, to care, to try, to step out, to step up, to put one's self on the line. *Why bother?*

The Six Ps of Progress – Pleasure

So if you got game, show it, share it. Spice it up. Be thrilling. Have some gusto. Dare to care. Truly care that the people who help you are receiving pleasure in the relationship.

Are you fond of those around you? Fake it and see what happens. I bet they become people you're fond of.

Show others the zest you have for your work. Zest offers pleasure.

No zest? Find it, create it, or move on.
Life is too short.

I could go on and on about pleasure, but as Stendhal (a complex and highly original French writer back in the 19th century) wrote, *"Pleasure is often spoiled by describing it."* I hope I didn't spoil anything for you.

Offer the Promise of Pleasure.

Be Progress.

For a solid example of offering the Promise of Pleasure, please see
The Way of the Donut Man
at the beginning of this book.

The Six Ps of Progress – Pleasure

The Way of the Donut Man, Revisited

I went back more than a year later to get the Donut Man's name and background for this book, and he remembered our brief conversation. His name is Inlark Han. He and his wife, Yoon, immigrated to the United States in 2001, along with their children, Jaeyoung and Seongmee, for their children's education. They bought an established donut shop, Sonny Donuts, in Allen, Texas, around that same time.

Inlark got the idea for the big blue umbrella after watching customers battle the rain to come into his store. Being in a shopping center, Sonny Donuts does not have a drive-thru. Inlark knew that when it rains, his customers could easily visit one of the several nearby competitors' drive-thrus to avoid getting wet.

To show his appreciation, Inlark quickly went out and bought the big blue umbrella and a poncho. (He was not wearing the poncho when we met.) Besides baking awesome (read: not oily) donuts and being a top-notch umbrella man, Inlark makes a point of greeting each customer by name when they visit. With her upbeat attitude, lively eyes, and enormous smile, Yoon is a big hit with customers as well.

Neither let their limited English intimidate them. Yoon says, *"We may not speak English well, but we try and we smile. And many customers want to learn some Korean too. That is nice."*

The Six Ps of Progress – Pleasure

Sonny Donuts is open seven days a week, from 5:00 a.m. until noon. Inlark and Yoon start baking each day at 1:30 a.m. They try to go to bed between 8:00 and 9:00 each night. Their busiest day is Saturday, with Sunday a close second.

Customers (including me) rave about their kolaches (pigs in a blanket to us Southern folk) because they are light and tasty. The glazed and chocolate donuts are also fantastic and big sellers as well.

In their few hours of free time, Inlark enjoys golf and Yoon explores her creativity by making the beautiful Korean paper crafts that decorate the walls of the donut shop. We all need creativity in our lives.

Sonny Donuts
1314 W. McDermott Drive, #145
Allen, Texas
972-359-0033

Tell them Dean sent you.

Ponder & Progress: The Pleasure 10

1. How do you, your services, your ideas, your products, your leadership style, your business plan and culture offer others pleasure?

2. Is there pleasure to be gained from working with you and for you? Oh, yeah? Like what?

3. How can you and your organization be better positioned as Agents of Pleasure in the minds of those you wish to inspire to action?

4. What pleasure do you get from your work?

5. How is accomplishing the goals you are committed to going to bring you pleasure?

6. How is working toward your goals bringing you pleasure?

7. How can you help coworkers, employees, and customers feel more pleasure in their work – and in their working relationship with you?

8. What aspects of your life and business should you improve to gain more pleasure?

9. How is your customer service (internal and external) a catalyst for others to feel pleasure?

10. How do you offer the Promise of Pleasure?

Profit

Most of us think "revenue" when we think profit. Therefore, it is helpful to include the terms *money* and *sales* when discussing the concept of feeling profit. *"Nothing happens until someone sells something"* is a dead-on classic business truism. On some level, we are ALL in sales. A job interview is a sales call; so is a date. We all sell something – our leadership, our action plan, our company, our old refrigerator. Sales is NOT a dirty word. Selling is the art of influence and attraction; so is business.

Sure, profit means *dinero* (Spanish for money), *geld* (German for money), and *pengar* (Swedish for money). But profit can also mean to prosper, to gain an advantage, or to improve. I even learned while doing research for this book that the word *profit* comes from a Latin word meaning "to make progress." *Cool, huh?*

So much of life is perception: perceived benefits, perceived value, and perceived profit. Prospects and customers need to perceive through our guidance and education that our product or service will fill their needs, meet their requirements, help them profit. Coworkers and employees need to perceive that the organization they work for (partner with) is heading in a direction that will be profitable for them.

The promise of profit helps form expectations. To encourage customer loyalty, quality referrals, and even productivity and employee retention, we must exceed expectations or at least match them.

The Six Ps of Progress – Profit

So, what do customers expect?
Everyone is different, but we can assume we all want quality products, a positive work environment, truly solid and caring customer service, even on-time delivery. We also want the products and services a sales professional recommends to actually be in our best interests and not just what the company is pushing this week, or those with the best profit margin.

> **"Profit is the celebration of service."**
> *-- Denis Waitley*

Customers, employees, and coworkers must believe they gain an upper hand in some way from their relationship with us and our companies. They must believe they profit from us, just as we are profiting from them.

Offer the Promise of Profit.

Be Progress.

The Origin of Upper Hand

The expression "upper hand" comes from America's once-favorite pastime, baseball. To decide which team would bat first in a sandlot baseball game, one player would grab a baseball bat at its base. A player from the other team would then place his hand above the first player's hand. Up the bat they would go, each gripping the bat until they reached the top. The player with the topmost hand would then have the "upper hand," with the choice of batting first.

The Way of a BAM
Becoming a Business Attraction Magnet

The business of sales is the business of attraction. We are attracted to products, services, ideas, and people that we trust can help us progress. Everyone profits when sales professionals focus on being progress, and being progress turns sales professionals into *Business Attraction Magnets*.

The great Dottie Walters, one of the founders of the National Speakers Association, shared with me many years ago that the word sales comes from the Scandinavian root word meaning to serve. Soak that in…**to serve**.

If we just made that little shift in our own thinking about that word *sales*, think of how many more people we could serve with our products, services, ideas, and contacts. (Not to mention our smiles and solid listening skills.) To sell is to serve. To serve is to *Be Progress*.

The days of the *"Surefire Closing Statement"* and the *"Glad-handing Slick Salesman"* are long gone. Today it is imperative for Progress Agents to truly get to know their prospects and help prospects get to know them. Selling is therefore a state of mind more than a series of steps. It is a dance, a buzz, a willingness to be involved, to connect, to attract. Those of us who make our careers selling are, by and large, outgoing, caring, and driven. We want to help others progress. We believe we can make a difference, that we can help. **Being progress puts wind in our sails and in our sales.**

The Six Ps of Progress – Profit

Becoming a Business Attraction Magnet is about trust. The customer has a need, or a step they desire to take. They must trust we can meet that need and help them take that step. Customers and prospects need to trust our belief in ourselves, in our companies, and in our products and services.

Seven Keys to Being a BAM

1. Become Buzz-worthy.
Business Attraction Magnets provide so much value, so much heat, and so much enthusiasm that customers are inspired to talk about them. A BAM is worthy of attention, worthy of the spotlight, worthy of wattage, and worthy of referrals.

As Progress Agents, we must not only show enthusiasm for our work – we must HAVE enthusiasm for our work. If we want prospects to get excited about our products and services, we need to have that excitement first. Likewise, if we want others to believe in our products and services, we must believe in our products and services first.

To win the prize, we must *be* the prize. Enthusiasm shows in the way we hold ourselves and in the passion we have for our jobs and our lives. If we want loyal customers and referrals *(and we do),* then we need to feel worthy of loyal customers and referrals. I am sure you have sensed by now that, whenever possible, people do business with people they like. Passion for our lives and belief in our work make us attractive and likable. They draw people to us. In sales, we have got to be *on*. Have game. Bring heat. Same is true for customer-service professionals and those in leadership. Buzz. Buzz.

The Six Ps of Progress – Profit

2. Ask Progress-Based, Open-Ended Questions.
In the medical profession, it is known that prescription without diagnosis is malpractice. The same is true for Business Attraction Magnets. We must ask a variety of open-ended questions to diagnose the situation, so our recommendation (prescription) will meet the need.

> **"The art and science of asking questions is the source of all knowledge."**
> *-- Thomas Berger*

There is a classic story, told in sales circles, of the inept salesman trying to explain to his boss why he closed only one sale per month. *"You know, you can lead a horse to water, but you can't make him drink,"* the salesman says, shrugging his shoulders. *"Make him drink?"* the manager replies. *"Your job is to make him thirsty."* That sounds good enough, but there's a fundamental oversight here: Clients and prospects are **already "thirsty."** They are thirsty for peace of mind, pleasure, profit, prestige, pain avoidance, and power. They are thirsty for progress. We must uncover others' particular parameters for progress if we hope to make them thirsty for the progress we offer.

The most powerful way to uncover the prospect's parameters for progress is to ask open-ended questions. These questions commonly include the basics of:
- Who
- What
- Where
- Why
- When
- How

The Six Ps of Progress – Profit

A BAM Dozen: 12 Solid Open-Ended Questions

Please find your own voice when asking these questions. We must be truly interested in finding a way to help.

1. *How* did you get interested in your line of work?
2. If a journalist were to write about what's been happening in your industry over the past six months, *what* might they write?
3. I connect with new people all the time; *how* would I know if someone qualified as a solid contact for you?
4. *How* would you define progress for you/your business?
5. *What* major shifts do you foresee in your industry?
6. *Where* do you see your greatest challenges?
7. *Why* do these challenges persist?
8. *What* difficulties will you face if you don't meet these challenges?
9. *What* actions are you taking to overcome these challenges?
10. *What* results are you expecting?
11. *Who* is involved in the decision-making process?
12. If you could solve these challenges, *what* kind of progress would you make?

Also, encourage prospects and clients to expand on their answers by asking:
    Would you tell me more about that?
    Could you please elaborate?
    Could you clarify...?
    How so?
    What did you mean when you said...?

Do not ask too many questions or ask them at a rocket-fire clip. People should not feel they are being interrogated. Being interrogated is neither attractive nor enjoyable.

3. Listen as if your lifestyle depended on it... *It Does!*
Solid listening goes hand in hand with asking powerful questions. I don't mean "listen" as in taking in sounds and passively processing them. As BAMs, we must LISTEN with all we've got. This is a basic but sometimes challenging principle to consistently put into practice. It means that, for the duration of our contact, we step outside of ourselves – our own needs, our every preconception – and attend entirely to someone else.

Everyone has a need to talk and be heard. Listening helps us treat others as if they were the most important people on the planet because – in their minds – they *are*. Many professionals forget to involve the prospect and drone on about how great their ideas or their company is, forgetting to ask probing questions and listening for ways to show how they can be progress for the other person.

Sometimes our motivation to actively listen is not all that high. We think we can get by without really focusing. This is a huge mistake. The ability to understand and value what others say is critical to being a BAM. So be determined to focus on and understand completely what others are trying to communicate. It is close to impossible to uncover someone's parameters of progress when you're preoccupied with previous conversations, unfinished tasks, or the impression you're making. Good listeners absorb and reflect on what they hear. They are active in the listening process. This requires energy and motivation, because listening is more than just hearing. We must become active listeners rather than passive hearers.

Repeating back (as questions or tentative statements) what you think you've heard the other person say helps avoid

The Six Ps of Progress – Profit

mind-misreading errors. Good clarifying questions offer the person a chance to rephrase their thoughts and say precisely what they mean.

4. Respect Time and Structure.
Structure is vital for becoming a *Business Attraction Magnet*. Solid self-management (*formerly known as time management: Tips on p. 145*) leads to higher productivity and reduced stress. Our desks need to be workstations, not storage space. We must be able to quickly locate important information. Being well organized shows a respect for time (ours and our customers').

Looking sharp is also part of solid organization. If we can't get ourselves together well enough to look presentable, *how are we going to be able to help someone else see us as together enough to handle their challenges?* Plus, how we present ourselves shouts volumes about how we feel about ourselves and our work. Becoming a Business Attraction Magnet takes preparation. Unfortunately, far too many of us invest more energy in planning our weekends, or even what we'll have for dinner, than we do our opportunities to be progress for prospects and customers.

Don't believe anyone who says sales is "just a numbers game." Sales is a Progress-based Impressions Game – a Proof-of-Progress Game – The Ultimate Game of Trust. Sure, the more contacts you make the better your odds – but you may also be blowing your chances for many potential relationships, not to mention time (yours and the prospect's), by rushing through the process half-cocked with an indifferent attitude. **The worst time to think of what you're going to say is as it's coming out of your mouth.**

The Six Ps of Progress – Profit

Ponder & Progress: Sales & Organization

Consider your three most recent sales presentations or sales phone calls:

1. Did you check your attitude before making contact?

2. Did you have a specific objective for the contact?

3. Did you have some ideas to offer on how you could Be Progress?

4. What was your plan?

5. Did you know what you were going to say?

6. Did you do enough research?

7. Did you set an appointment?

8. Were your materials in order?

9. Were your questions relevant and helpful?

10. Was the person inspired to positive action?

<u>Bonus Question:</u>
Did you make a sale or start a progress-based relationship?

Prepare, keep your enthusiasm, and be persistent. Eighty percent of new sales are made on the fifth contact, yet the majority of salespeople give up after the second contact. Give full attention to every relationship opportunity. Being well organized makes it easier to build trust and offer progress.

5. Build Priceless Business Relationships

I wrote a whole book on building priceless business relationships so I'm not going to rewrite it here. But I will say this: Building priceless business relationships does NOT hinge on who we know, or even who knows us. The key to building priceless business relationships is to proactively use what we know about who we know so that we can position ourselves as progress in the minds of those we wish to build priceless business relationships with.

I know I rolled through that rather quickly and wordily. For more information on building priceless business relationships, I strongly encourage you to check out *Cracking the Networking CODE: 4 Steps to Priceless Business Relationships* by Dean Lindsay. I could not recommend this gentleman's work more highly (and he is so humble). But I digress...

6. Practice Empathy.

Empathy is knowing and feeling where the other person is coming from, walking a mile in their shoes, seeing things from their point of view. Empathy involves understanding that people make decisions for their own reasons, not ours. There are always reasons. Customers have reasons, prospects have reasons, employees have reasons, coworkers have reasons. They might not be our reasons.

To enhance our level of empathy, it is paramount to focus on understanding others' parameters for progress. We may never fully uncover where another person's motivation, their *"motives for actions,"* are coming from, but those motives, along with their parameters for progress, are uniquely theirs.

The Six Ps of Progress – Profit

To be a Business Attraction Magnet, always think, and say: *"What that means to you, Mrs./Mr. Prospect, is…"* Commit to doing what is best for the customer, ever striving to help provide the right product or service to meet their needs. Sure, we want to profit, but the customer's profit is key to ours. Practicing empathy includes understanding that customers do not want our products and services – they want what they think our products and services can do for them.

One of my client companies is among the largest trade show booth manufacturers in the USA. They design, build, and transport the huge trade show booths you see at the big conferences around the country and world. At the very beginning of a program I was conducting for their sales teams, I stated bluntly, *"No one wants a trade booth."*

The room went silent. The reps looked at the Vice President of Sales and each other as if to say, *"What?"*
Finally, one of the sales managers in the back raised his hand and said, *"No, Dean. They actually call us up and order trade show booths."*
I said, *"You bet. They order trade show booths, but a trade show booth is not really what they want."*
Again more silence. Then the Vice President of Sales spoke. *"You're right, Dean. Our customers don't want trade show booths – they want profit. We must be able to show them how investing in our trade show booths will help them to profit."*

Business Attraction Magnets know it is not the goal of having the product or service itself that creates the momentum. It is the perceived benefits (feelings realized) behind having or utilizing the product or service that creates the momentum.

The Six Ps of Progress – Profit

7. Focus on Value and Cost, Not Price.
Sure, it is easy for prospects, as well as sales professionals, to focus on price because it's right there in black and white. And true, our products and services do come with a price. But the _price_ of a product or service isn't what the product or service actually _costs_. We must show that every penny of the price is necessary, because it offers the best _value_ and avoids the cost of alternative purchases and situations. Cost and value are hard to nail down but are far more important figures to relate – because they include not only the price, but also the value-added service, technical support, our expertise, and all the other progress-based aspects that go along with a relationship with us and our company. There are often ramifications from purchasing-decisions that are eventually felt within other departments. True value shows itself over time. The challenge and responsibility of a sales professional is to relay the true costs of other choices upfront. Buyers must see that they profit by investing their time and money with us.

"Our prices are too high" is often the excuse heard from sales professionals as they explain their less-than-stellar sales performance. Sometimes it's true. Most of the time, however, the issue is not our price; it's articulating the true cost, and how working with us and agreeing to our price is the best value option and therefore means progress. If prospects have a strong enough why, they will figure out the how. If employees have a strong enough why, they too will figure out the how. When things get tough, reminding coworkers, employees, and ourselves of the progress behind the desired actions is paramount.

Become a *Business Attraction Magnet*. Offer the Promise of Profit. Be Progress.

Ponder and Progress: The Profit 10

1. How do you, your services, your ideas, your products, your leadership style, your business plan and culture offer others profit?

2. Is there profit to be gained from working with you and for you? Oh, yeah? Like what?

3. How can you and your organization be better positioned as Agents of Profit in the minds of those you wish to inspire to action?

4. How can you help all involved focus on <u>cost</u>, not price?

5. How is accomplishing the goals you are committed to going to bring you profit?

6. How is working toward your goals bringing you profit?

7. How do you profit from better teamwork and by helping your company profit and become more productive?

8. What aspects of your life and business should you improve to gain more profit?

9. How is your customer service (internal and external) a catalyst for others to feel they are profiting?

10. How do you offer the Promise of Profit?

<u>Bonus Question to Ponder:</u> How are you attracting and retaining customers in this tough economy and competitive market?

Prestige

We all want dignity, to feel we have the esteem of others, to feel that we are important and have influence. Few of us wish to live in obscurity or feel insignificant, and no one wants to feel mediocre. Prestige is the level of respect at which one is regarded by others.

Distinction can bring prestige. Awards, such as the Nobel, an Oscar, Employee of the Month, Customer of the Month, and MVP can elevate our standing in the eyes of others. Prizes also offer prestige. Sales awards offer prestige. *And what do many sales reps do after they win an annual sales award?* They win it again next year, or get darn close!

It is natural to want some proof of achievement, some way to look back and simply show someone what we did. My elder daughter, Sofia, feels prestige from earning her black belt in Tang Soo Do; younger daughter, Ella, feels prestige from the kudos she gets on her art projects and witty rhyming. Heck, I still have my Little League baseball trophies *(I'm not presently displaying them but I might, and I sure did back in the day)*.

For wins and grins, be ears and cheers. Sharing the credit leads to more credit to share. Give kudos. Prominence is good in the right doses. A little deserved fame can start a progress flame. We could all use a pat on the back. And it feels just as good to give someone else's back a pat. As Samuel Goldwyn, the G in MGM, said, *"When someone does something good, applaud! You will make two people happy."* Get a boost from being the boost.

The Six Ps of Progress – Prestige

Help people feel they have game, and help them celebrate that game. The recognition does not have to be complicated or even have an earth-shattering "WOW" factor. One of my favorite restaurants, The Bavarian Grill (BavarianGrill.com) in Plano, Texas, does something cool enough and it's simple.

They created a Stein Club that offers patrons the opportunity to earn a stein (ceramic beer mug) with the patron's name emblazoned on it. The patrons have their choice of taking their personalized stein home or having it hang on the walls of the Bavarian Grill's Biergärten (beer garden). Most choose the second option and feel some prestige in having a stein with their name on it displayed in the beer garden. (I know I do.)

However, I am not only talking about awards. Praise works, too. Compliments can offer prestige and a mental leg up. Express a <u>sincere</u> compliment, even on little stuff.
"I like your hair."
"Cool shoes."
"Good show."

> **"Praise can be your most valuable asset as long as you don't aim it at yourself."**
> -- *O.A. Battista*

Offer the promise of prestige. Be Progress.

<u>The Origin of a Leg Up:</u>
Our idiom "leg up" comes from receiving help when getting on a horse. Someone cups their hands, the rider puts his or her foot in there, and the helper lifts the rider up as the rider throws the other leg up and over the horse.

The Six Ps of Progress – Prestige

The Name Game

Something as simple as remembering and using people's names offers prestige. Everybody wants to feel the prestige of being thought of as unique, memorable, and important. A person's name is as important to them as yours is to you. Unfortunately, too many professionals have shared with me that they <u>can't remember</u> names. I'll ask, *"You mean you meet someone one day and then you see them three weeks later and can't remember their name?"*

"No," they answer. *"People introduce themselves. I introduce myself, and then... poof! The name disappears."* I do not think that in these cases we actually have trouble remembering names. I don't think we truly <u>heard</u> the name in the first place. To be able to offer the prestige that comes from using someone's name, make a point of catching and then tossing the name around in conversation. Here is a four-step process for remembering names.

The Name Game
1. Right before you meet new people, focus. Prepare to catch their name. If you do not catch it, ask them to repeat it rather than letting it go. Do not be embarrassed to ask. (They probably did not catch your name, either.)
2. Casually toss their name back in your first or second response.
3. Mention their name naturally throughout the conversation but DO NOT overuse it.
4. Repeat their name when parting.

Offer the Promise of Prestige. Be Progress.

The Way of the Compliment

> "Everybody likes a compliment."
> -- Abraham Lincoln

A sincere compliment is a great way to offer the promise of prestige. Sincere compliments cost us nothing yet can become priceless for both the giver and receiver. As Mark Twain wrote, *"I can live for two months on a good compliment."* Also consider that compliments can be used as conversation starters when we add progress based open-ended questions that relate to the compliment.

It takes some confidence to notice good things about others and to tell them about it. Giving people a lift has the power of raising our confidence even further because when we start noticing good things about people, we often start noticing more good things about ourselves also. But be careful, compliments that are ill-timed or thought to be insincere are likely to have the opposite effect than intended. *Here are four and a half quick tips:*

1. Practice <u>sincerely</u> complimenting others.
Start by finding something, however small, to genuinely praise others for. The more specific the better because it shows the person we truly noticed them.

2. Personalize the compliment.
Take the person's interests into account. When communicating with someone, be on the alert for traits they value in themselves. Personalized compliments can go a long way in offering prestige but it's best not to use them to often on the same person for they might be considered fake.

The Six Ps of Progress - Prestige

3. Share Others' compliments.
No, I don't mean bragging about good stuff people have said about you. I mean share the good stuff you have heard about others. A weird thing about us humans is that often when we hear bad things we are quick to tell others, but when hear anything nice about somebody else, we often keep it to ourselves. *Bad form humans.* When we hear something nice about someone, we need to share it with the person being complimented. They are likely to feel prestige from hearing it, and a bit of that Progress lands right on us.

4. Imply the compliment.
Often, we assume more truth from things we figure out for ourselves, than from facts handed to us. Try letting the intended recipient use their inner 'Sherlock Holmes' by allowing them to deduce the compliment from your comments. By indirectly complimenting we offer the promise of prestige, while avoiding sounding like a flatterer. *"Wow, you finished college in three years, it took me four and a half"* might carry more weight than *"You're smarter and more focused than me"*.

4 ½. Explain the compliment.
Instead of implying, try the opposite. Compliments can also become stronger when we share the why behind the compliment. *"That color looks good on you because it matches your eyes."*

> **"If people did not compliment one another there would be little society."**
> -- Marquis De Vauvenargues

Offer the Promise of Prestige.

Be Progress.

The Six Ps of Progress - Prestige

Ponder and Progress: The Prestige 10

1. How do you, your services, your ideas, your products, your leadership style, your business plan and culture offer others prestige?

2. Is there prestige to be gained from working with you and for you? Oh, yeah? Like what?

3. How can you and your organization be better positioned as Agents of Prestige in the minds of those you wish to inspire to action?

4. How important is prestige to you? To your team members? To your customers?

5. How is accomplishing the goals you are committed to going to bring you prestige?

6. How is working toward your goals bringing you prestige?

7. How can you help encourage and inspire coworkers and employees by offering prestige for accomplishing individual and team goals?

8. What prestige is there for customers in giving referrals to you and your business?

9. How do your products and services help customers and clients gain recognition for their life and business?

10. How do you offer the Promise of Prestige?

Pain Avoidance

Wow, we have an awful lot of words for pain: *Disappointment, Despair, Cramp, Torment, Regret, Stress, Worry, Irritation, Shock, Woundedness, Affliction, Bother, Agony, Suffering, Bitterness, Distress, Headache, Heartache, Grief, Crick, Sting, Hurt, Punishment, Misery, Aversion, Harm, Disgust, Ache, Discomfort, Trouble, Sadness, Anxiety, Tribulation, Woe, Distaste, Unpleasantness, Annoyance, Boredom, Drag, Anguish, Nuisance.*

We have darting pain, sharp pain, shooting pain. Pain can be physical (nausea, sore back, an itch) or mental (anxiety, hatred, even boredom). We each feel pain during our lives. The feeling of pain is one of the main factors that organize meaning in our world and psyche. Therefore, pain avoidance is a key pursuit.

> **"Pain is meant to wake us up."**
> *--Jim Morrison*

Social services, humanitarian aid, public-health initiatives, community development, economic aid, human rights programs, disaster relief, and pretty much all forms of philanthropy are all ways to help people avoid, prevent, or relieve pain. Scientists work to end disease, parents pass down tools to their children for coping with life's challenges, musicians even write songs that help take our minds off our daily worries and thus avoid pain.

The Six Ps of Progress – Pain Avoidance

A good health-benefits package is a pain-avoidance package. Good fire departments, the right pair of shoes, and toothpaste with fluoride all offer pain avoidance. So do homes in safe neighborhoods, foods with low LDL cholesterol, vehicles with anti-lock brakes, vitamins, exercise equipment, and good mortgage rates. Well-trained, highly motivated, and professionally led armed forces offer pain avoidance via the same dynamics as a well-trained, highly motivated, and professionally led customer-service department. And the list goes on.

The marketing campaigns for many everyday products are built around encouraging us to view the products as solid ways to avoid pain. Consider Calgon bath products, for example. Their slogan is: *Take Me Away*. Their website is even TakeMeAway.com.

Away from what?
Away from our stresses, away from our pressures, away from pain. We all have escape mechanisms or strategies for avoiding unpleasantness.

Why do people avoid an annoying or troublesome whiner or blowhard? Because they are painful to be around. (Heck, we even call them a "pain in the neck.")

"Pain leadership" and punitive pain-parenting are, unfortunately, common motivational strategies. Being grounded, no iPod for a month, a dock in pay, and the risk of being fired are all ways of communicating: *If you want to avoid pain, do what I want you to do*! Reminders of past pain serve as motivators as well. Coaches show players footage of a painful team defeat to inspire them to play their best so they won't feel the agony of defeat again.

The Six Ps of Progress – Pain Avoidance

We all want to avoid pain, but often we don't fully consider the consequences of actions or inactions that will be painful in the long term.

What is more painful to you: Self-Discipline or Regret?

If we can feel the future pain now in enough detail, then we will be compelled to do everything and anything to avoid that pain in the future – i.e., we will work toward achieving the goal. Sometimes choosing to go through pain is smart, but it still smarts. Paying our insurance premium is not painless, but most would agree that not having insurance would be more painful.

> "And there ain't nothing like regret to remind you you're alive."
> *-- Sheryl Crow*

Prospecting, dealing with demanding customers, or getting up to speed on new company products can be painful. But there is also pain in not prospecting, not dealing with demanding customers, and not getting up to speed on new company products.

Each individual's attitude toward pain varies greatly, depending on whether the person deems the pain useless or useful, unavoidable or avoidable, unacceptable or acceptable, even undeserved or deserved. Unmet needs stay painfully in mind. Unmet potential can be painful, too. There is pain in leaving the status quo for the unknown, in risk-taking. Therefore, it can be painful to progress.

The Six Ps of Progress – Pain Avoidance

Some risks are worth taking, others not. Each of us gets to decide. As Progress Agents, we should be able to show prospects and coworkers (as well as ourselves) how there is more pain in not going through the pain of leaving the status quo, more pain in avoiding the unknown, more pain in the risk not taken.

Offer the Promise of Pain Avoidance.

Be Progress.

The Six Ps of Progress – Pain Avoidance

The Way of
the Entrepreneurial Drill Sergeant

For many years, I facilitated a goal-commitment program that I created, called Big PHAT Goals. PHAT is a hip-hop slang acronym that stands for Pretty, Hot, And Tempting. Basically, PHAT means attractive. Our goals have to be attractive to us if we are going to be committed to them. Our products and services have to be attractive to clients and prospects if they are going to commit their money and time. Likewise, our ideas and initiatives have to be attractive to those we'd like to see involved in their implementation.

Once early in my career, after presenting a speech on goal commitment to a group of area business owners, I caught the eye of an extremely fit man standing ramrod straight and tall. Sporting a crew cut, polished army boots, camouflage pants, and a dark green monogrammed T-shirt, he really stood out (not your normal attire for this type of function).

We nodded to each other and I could tell by his body language that he was waiting for the right moment to come speak with me. After several other participants and I had discussed my speech and some opportunities, the gentleman walked up to me, coming to a stop just a little closer to me than was normal. In a commanding but not loud voice he said, *"Dean?"*
I responded, almost instinctively, *"Yes, sir!"*
He said, *"I've got a military background."*
I said, *"Yes, sir. I could tell, sir."*

The Six Ps of Progress – Pain Avoidance

He said, *"Drill sergeant, eight years. I now run a fitness boot camp. Good speech. I'd like to have you present your Big PHAT program to my cadets next Saturday."*

At this point in my business career I did not need to check my calendar. *"Yes, sir."*

He continued, *"Why don't you come by next Tuesday evening? We can discuss the program and I'll give you a tour of the campus. You'll get a chance to meet some of the cadets and we can get them worked up about the workshop."* *"Yes, sir,"* I said. Again, no calendar required.

He told me he had rented some warehouse space on the outskirts of town for his campus, and that his cadets arrived at 5:40 p.m. and drills started at 6:00 p.m. sharp. I arrived at his place that next Tuesday at 5:15 p.m.

I walked into what seemed like a normal office. He greeted me and spent several minutes discussing why he was interested in the workshop. The drill sergeant shared his desire to help his cadets reach their fitness goals, and that he believed the Big PHAT Goals program could help. He understood that each of us commits to a goal with strong reasons and the best of intentions. But without constant reinforcement, our strong reasons can weaken over time to the point where some other action becomes more attractive.

We discussed how each of us is continuously motivated to do one thing or another (get up, sleep in. Eat the cheesecake, not eat the cheesecake). Consciously or subconsciously, we are constantly deciding that some outcomes are more attractive or more tempting than others, and we act accordingly.

The Six Ps of Progress – Pain Avoidance

I could relate. For decades, I had the habit of setting a New Year's resolution to lose weight. Each year I would get myself a fitness membership and work out a few times, only to stumble back into my "normal" routine. I never forgot that I wanted to be skinny, but I did lose sight of why I wanted to be skinny. There were so many other things that I could choose to do with that time.

As we talked, I quickly realized the drill sergeant caught the concept of using the Six Ps of Progress to propel action. He understood that we needed to help his cadets truly internalize the reasons behind their movements and offer them tools to help them stay committed to their goals.

"Dean, let me show you the campus," he said.
"Yes, sir." I had been wondering about this campus.
He opened up the back door to the office, revealing a long thin room with a concrete floor and a metal roof. Calling the sarge's campus "old school" would be a stretch. I doubt he had invested more than seventy-five dollars outfitting the whole place. He had drilled holes in the concrete walls and stuck in metal poles for pull-ups. Concrete blocks with twine handles served for curls, and sheets of cardboard in one corner marked the spot where cadets did their sit-ups and their push-ups. He'd even mowed a half-mile running track though the fields and woods behind the warehouse (I mean, *campus*). This was definitely not Life Time Fitness.

I was really curious about what type of people were enrolled in the drill sergeant's boot camp. Then they started to arrive. They were regular people! Good, solid, hardworking folks (like us); a few still had their badges on from the places where they worked. And he treated them like normal people, until the first one came out of the changing room wearing

The Six Ps of Progress – Pain Avoidance

bright orange shorts and a gray shirt. (Turns out everyone had matching bright orange shorts and gray shirts. Pause a second to get the visual.)

When the last cadet came out in her attire, the drill sergeant reached into the bottom drawer of his desk and pulled out his drill sergeant hat, one of those *Smokey the Bear Meets Full Metal Jacket* hats with the hard brim that goes all the way around.

As soon as the hat hit his head, his intensity went to 11. He barked, *"All right. Let's go, grunts!"* and in a flash, they all ran out the back door to the track. About ten minutes later, the drill sergeant marched his cadets back in. Each was breaking a pretty decent sweat. Meanwhile, the sergeant was still barking orders, now mixed with song lyrics: *"Pick up that concrete, put it down. Go over there and give me fifteen. Gotta get up to get down, my little grunts. Gotta get up to get down. Chin up!"*

This guy was a trip. He got right up in their faces, then suddenly yelled, *"Grunts to the mat and sit!"*
They knew exactly what that meant. The cadets all scrambled over to the cardboard and sat down, Indian style. They were panting and wiping sweat from their eyes. After pacing in front of them for about a minute, he waved me over. *"C'mon over here, big PHAT guy."*

I know what you're thinking: "Big PHAT Guy" – not a great moniker. But hey, it's branding, and at that point in my career I was glad to be known as anything. So I was the Big PHAT guy. *"Come over here, Big PHAT guy. Tell us about your awesome program to help my cadets stick to their guns."*

The Six Ps of Progress – Pain Avoidance

As I walked over to them, I could have sworn I saw a couple of them mouth, *"Thank you"* to me for getting them a break. I did not aspire to match the drill sergeant's presentation style, so I asked plainly, with little emotion, *"How many of you are here to avoid pain?"*

The cadets looked confused by the question and no one raised their hand. They were in pain. Couldn't I see that? How could they be going through this boot camp to avoid pain? I asked again, *"How many are here to avoid pain?"*

The drill sergeant raised his hand. I said, *"Yes, sir?"* He said, *"My cadets are here to avoid pain – let there be no doubt. My cadets feel pain in not being able to fit into anything in their closet, not being able to walk up a flight and a half of stairs without huffing and puffing. Some even worry about dying from a heart pain before their kids graduate from high school. My painful boot camp helps them avoid that pain."* The cadets stared at the drill sergeant for a few seconds and then, one by one, each started nodding in agreement. I could see a sense of purpose build in their eyes. They were there to avoid pain.

The Big PHAT Goals program the following Saturday was well attended, and every one of the drill sergeant's "grunts" participated (maybe they were scared not to). The cadets made lists of the pain they were working to avoid by being in the boot camp. Items included diabetes, joint and back pain, personal disappointment, and loneliness. Though the program was many years ago, one of the drill sergeant's grunts recently contacted me to share that she still reads over her list to keep herself attracted to her fitness goals.

Offer the Promise of Pain Avoidance. Be Progress.

Ponder & Progress: The Pain Avoidance 10

1. How do you, your services, your ideas, your products, your leadership style, your business plan and culture offer others pain avoidance?

2. Is there pain to be avoided by working with you and for you? Oh, yeah? Like what?

3. How can you and your organization be better positioned as Agents of Pain Avoidance in the minds of those you wish to inspire to action?

4. What is more painful to you – <u>self-discipline</u> or <u>regret</u>?

5. How is accomplishing the goals you are committed to going to help you avoid pain?

6. How is working toward your goals helping you avoid pain?

7. How can you better share how you offer pain avoidance to prospects, clients, and customers?

8. What aspects of your life and business should you improve to help you avoid pain?

9. How does your customer service (internal and external) help others to avoid pain?

10. How do you offer the Promise of Pain Avoidance?

The Six Ps of Progress – Power

Power

When considering the meaning of power, many words come to mind: *clout, brawn, capacity, ability, might, influence, muscle, steam, horsepower, leadership.* But the word that sums up the true feeling of power is the word **Choice**, the power to determine our own thoughts and actions.

Who has power? Everyone. Each of us has the power of choice. We each hold the power of decision making. Even self-discipline is flexing our power of choice *(mind over ice cream)*.

> **"A human being is a deciding being."**
> *-- Viktor Frankl*

Power is not just enforcement. In the form of influence and persuasion, power is used in countless ways to encourage people to choose to act, feel, and behave in ways other than how they may have initially planned, or would habitually react. Each of us would make different choices if we were influenced differently. In essence, all human interaction involves power, because ideas hold power, and ideas underlie all language and action.

There is power in branding. There is power in marketing, in PR, in advertising. There is power in "word of mouth" and in social influence. There is power in shared beliefs. Expertise offers power. Training leads to power. Degrees can translate as power. Positions can hold power. Power is exercised when we are able to reward and promote. Wealth can bring power. Some feel power from being accepted.

The Six Ps of Progress – Power

Education offers the promise of power because it builds the mental qualities and knowledge to make choices that get things done. But it is not only knowledge that offers power; being able to communicate knowledge is also power. It is not just what we know or whom we know; it is mainly what we decide to DO with what we know that is paramount.

Power is the ability (present or anticipated) to make choices that bring about significant *change*, usually in people's lives, through one's own actions or those of others. *Nengli*, the Mandarin word for power, literally means "can-strength," or "being capable." To influence others, one must have some understanding and mastery of the situations or things the other person desires or needs. A boss, manager, or employer wields power over employees because he or she commonly controls projects, working conditions, wages, hiring and firing, etc. However, employees hold power, too. They can quit, slack off, form a union, steal pens and toilet paper, undermine coworkers' morale, provide lousy service, and be all-out liabilities. Employees can also arrive on time, be supportive team players, think outside of the box, and provide world-class service. It all comes down to the power of choice.

> **"Everything can be taken from a man but one thing: the last of the human freedoms – to choose one's attitude in any given set of circumstances, to choose one's own way."**
> -- *Viktor Frankl*

All parties in all relationships have some power. Customers have power to choose to spend their money wherever they please. Companies have the power to alter policies or refuse service. Power can be delegated, but only to those who choose to accept the power.

The Six Ps of Progress – Power

One primitive but common way of obtaining the feeling of power is by threatening someone with pain *(firing, a bonk on the head, no dessert)*. There is power in threatening pain. But this kind of thought and behavior is a negative misuse of power and is always counterproductive. As any student of world history or "office politics" will tell you, such "power" inevitably builds resentment and resistance. And, there is power in resistance. *"Fight the Power"* is itself a statement of power.

Someone's awareness of us and our abilities can have powerful results. People carry archives of knowledge and impressions within their gray matter, and it behooves us to have ourselves archived as a source of power. Powerful people are those with easy access to resources, those who can reliably exercise their will, their ideas, and their way. Progress Agents are able to show how the choices we want others to make will bring them more choices, more power, more progress. But it is still each individual's choice as to what to think and believe, and how to act.

> **"Between stimulus and response there is a space. In that space is our power to choose our response. In our response lies our growth and our freedom."**
> *-- Viktor Frankl*

Offer the promise of power.

Be Progress.

The Six Ps of Progress – Power

The Way of Viktor Frankl

Viktor Frankl, M.D., Ph.D. (1905-1997), was an Austrian neurologist, a Holocaust survivor, and one of the greatest European psychiatrists of the twentieth century. The U.S. Library of Congress named Dr. Frankl's enlightening masterpiece, *Man's Search for Meaning,* one of the 10 books that "made the most difference in people's lives."

Dr. Frankl is the founder of logotherapy, which he derived from the words: <u>logos</u> – Greek for *reason* or *meaning*, and *therapy* – Greek, meaning *I heal.* <u>Logotherapy</u> therefore means *"Reasons I heal" or "Healing the Meaning"* (trippy, profound, and enlightening both ways).

The basic philosophy of logotherapy is that people have a will to find meaning and that life can have meaning under all circumstances, even the most miserable. Each of us has the freedom, under all circumstances, to choose to find reasons to endure and progress.

> **"Ever more people today have the means to live, but no meaning to live for."**
> *-- Viktor Frankl*

We have freedom to find meaning in what we do and experience. We have freedom to take a stand when faced with an unjust and possibly unchangeable situation. We each have the power of choice to find our unique meaning in life. Frankl believed we all have more of a desire to *feel powerful* than to *obtain power* (and there is a big difference).

The Six Ps of Progress – Power

Frankl first used the term logotherapy in 1926, and had developed some of its basic tenets before he was sent to a Nazi concentration camp in 1942. He even had a manuscript devoted to his views sewn into the clothes he wore when he was sent there. However the Nazis found the manuscript, so Frankl's life's work went up in flames.

Frankl knew he had valuable ideas, but no way of actually sharing them with the world. Early on in his time in the camps he decided to recreate the manuscript, and did so on scraps of paper hidden from guards. He also used the harsh camp environment as his field study. Frankl worked passionately to prevent inmate suicide and alleviate gloom and depression in fellow prisoners. The Nazis did not allow anyone to actively intervene in an actual suicide attempt, so Frankl's efforts were preventative and kept secret.

He found that very few of his fellow inmates said, *"I want to die."* Most said that they wanted to live, but the ones who eventually survived the camps were those who had focused reasons attached to their survival wish – loved ones to reunite with, something to work for or to look forward to. Frankl theorized that when we have enough meaning attached to an outcome, we are able to withstand the suffering related to achieving it.

Frankl's meaning, his *strong reasons* for surviving, were connected not only to his hope of reuniting with his young wife Tilly, as well as his mother, father and brother, but also to his work. He wanted to survive, had to survive, partly because he had powerful and helpful beliefs about the human condition that he needed to recreate and share with the world.

The Six Ps of Progress – Power

Freed after three years at Auschwitz, Dachau, and other concentration camps, he returned to Vienna and began work on a book with the literal English translation: *From Death Camp to Existentialism: A Psychiatrist's Path to a New Therapy* (In the U.S, we call it *Man's Search for Meaning*.) In the book, Frankl describes *(from the unique perspective of a psychiatrist)* the horrific life of a concentration camp inmate. With this desire to feel autonomous and powerful, and to work and win in a world of change, we can benefit greatly from a look into Dr. Frankl's teachings.

Three Progress Action Steps from the Work of Dr. Frankl

1. Harness the Freedom of Choice.
As markets continue to fluctuate, business challenges mount, and personal issues multiply, we each have the freedom to choose our reaction. A resourceful attitude toward a challenge is essential if the challenge is to be met. Dr. Frankl's pregnant wife, his parents and brother were all killed during their incarceration in Nazi prison camps. He'd lost everything, he said, that could be taken from a person, except one thing: *"the last of the human freedoms, to choose one's attitude in any given set of circumstances, to choose one's own way."* We each have the power to choose, but that power is wasted if we do not exercise it.

In the face of inescapable uncertainty (i.e., business challenges, a slowing economy, stiff competition), we must fire up the unwavering determination that comes from possessing strong reasons to overcome our daily challenges. Frankl was a man of action. He believed we must act, must do, must persist.

2. Take Responsibility for Actions.
Frankl taught that life has an urgency to which people must respond if decisions are to be meaningful. Each of us must take responsibility for where we are in our financial situation, in our relationships, and in our career, because it is our decisions that put us there. We have the power of choice and are responsible for those choices. We have not only a right, but a responsibility, to fulfill our individual potential, according to Frankl.

> **"Life ultimately means taking the responsibility to find the right answers to its problems and to fulfill the tasks which it constantly sets for each individual."**
> -- *Viktor Frankl*

Frankl discovered that it is not what happens to us that matters. It is how we respond to what happens that is significant. Same with business. We cannot control all the elements of our personal life or business.
- Trucks break down.
- Water heaters burst.
- Computers crash (so do entire economies).
- Customers move.
- Kids get sick.
- Venders go out of business.
- Things happen.

The only things we can control are our responses, our decisions, our actions. Our actions are our responsibility.

3. Drive Actions by Understanding Goals and Strengths.
Gaining insight into a person's reasons *(especially our own)* goes a long way in helping them progress and reach their full potential. Frankl believed in endurance, but not just for the sake of survival.

He believed that all life is shot through with significance, and that this inherent meaningfulness should motivate humans to live and discover that meaning. Frankl warned that some may mistake the surface rewards of materialism, affluence, or hedonism as the true purpose of life.

Those who have suffered loss due to injustice (racial profiling, crime), circumstance (accidents, economy, acts of nature), or the inhumanity of fellow humans know that the search for meaning is not stopped by setbacks. In many cases, as in Frankl's, challenges and adversities serve to inspire and redirect a more determined search for meaning.

> **"Life can be pulled by goals just as surely as it can be pushed by drives."**
> *-- Viktor Frankl*

Great leaders understand the necessity of discovering what their followers are made of, what they're "all about." Frankl firmly believed in the great potential of his fellow humans, and stressed the ability to use one's inner resources to achieve personal goals and find personal truth. This principle applies equally to every organization. Each member, no matter the responsibility or position, has unique strengths that can prove vital in fueling the progress of the organization.

What drives the people you hope to inspire to action?

What drives you?

A few more Frankl Facts:

During his youth, he wrote to Sigmund Freud. After Freud replied, a lively correspondence developed. Viktor traveled extensively, enjoyed a lifelong passion for mountain climbing, and even obtained his pilot's license while in his sixties.

Dr. Frankl's awards and honors include the John F. Kennedy Star, the Albert Schweitzer Medal and the Oskar Pfister Award (the highest honor given by the American Psychiatric Association). He was even nominated for the Nobel Peace Prize.

Dr. Frankl wrote over 30 books, had over 700 scholarly articles published in the world's most prestigious scientific journals, and lectured at over 200 universities in more than 40 countries, on all seven continents. However, in his autobiography, Frankl writes, "In my view, I was never a big thinker. But one thing I may have been through my life: a thorough and persistent "thinker-through." (A thinker-through…I like that.) Viktor Frankl died of cardiac arrest on the 2nd of September, 1997, in Vienna, Austria, at the age of 92.

Viktor Frankl was Progress!

The Six Ps of Progress – Power

Ponder & Progress: The Power 10

1. How do you, your services, your ideas, your products, your leadership style, your business plan and culture offer others power?

2. Is there power to be gained from working with you and for you? Oh, yeah? Like what?

3. How can you and your organization be better positioned as Agents of Power in the minds of those you wish to inspire to action?

4. How will you remind yourself that you always have the power of choice even in uncomfortable or negative situations?

5. How is accomplishing the goals you are committed to going to bring you power?

6. How is working toward your goals bringing you power?

7. What in particular does your product or service enable people to do that they could not otherwise do?

8. What aspects of your life and business should you improve to gain more power?

9. How is your customer service (internal and external) a catalyst for others to feel powerful?

10. How do you offer the Promise of Power?

What about Pride and Purpose?

I considered whether I should add Pride and, to a lesser degree, Purpose to the Ps of Progress, and decided not to. Over the years, I have asked many friends and peers to describe *feeling pride,* and each has described a special combination of pleasure, peace of mind, and prestige – sometimes with a little pain avoidance, profit, and power thrown into the mix.

Pride may be a solid and realistic sense of one's dignity, value, and self-respect, but the word *pride* is also associated with feeling lofty, or making an arrogant assumption of superiority. *Pride* often has negative connotations, such as haughtiness, vanity, conceit, egoism, grandiosity, narcissism, being a braggart, and so on.

> **"Pride is pleasure arising from a man's thinking too highly of himself."**
> *-- Baruch Spinoza*

Excessive pride, according to the writings of Aristotle, is commonly the defining trait that leads to a hero's tragic downfall. Heck, pride is one of the Seven Deadly Sins! Pride is even commonly considered the original and most serious of the deadly sins – the source from which all others arise. In the story of Lucifer, pride was what caused his fall from heaven, and his transformation into Satan. This story alone shows that *Pride* can be a real downer. So, given its unhappy history, I felt it best that *Pride* not be included as one of the *Ps of Progress.*

The Six Ps of Progress

At the same time, the rightful feeling of pride – as in self-respect, or pride in one's work or the work of the team – is vital for progress. When people have little or no self-respect or pride in themselves or their work, they feel increasingly discouraged, powerless, and inferior.

So pride is tricky. Speaking of the inflated and distorted kind of pride, nineteenth-century author John Ruskin observed: *"In general, pride is at the bottom of all great mistakes."* A Hebrew proverb further admonishes: "Pride goes before a fall" – whether it's a dethroned monarch or the demoted John Q. Blowhard.

The term *purpose* generally holds different meanings for different people, but purpose is not a feeling. Purpose is the idea, the objective, the passion behind our actions. Our life's purpose is the core compelling force that pulls us forward. Purpose is direction with *meaning*. And we develop our meaning based upon what we believe will result in us feeling the *Six Ps of Progress*. Having a sense of purpose leads to our feeling the Six Ps of Progress.

How do you feel when you know and are following your purpose?

When is pride a negative for you?

The Six Ps of Progress

The Seven Deadly Sins, Visited or Revisited:

These failings, for anyone keeping score, are:
Lust, Gluttony, Greed, Sloth, Wrath, Envy, and Pride.
I sure wish I could share some personal examples of each sin but, to the best of my knowledge – or should I say memory – I have never personally committed any of them. (Stop laughing.)

The idea of Seven Deadly Sins was originally used by early Christian leaders to spotlight – and make people wary of – their tendency to sin. Around the 14th century, the Seven Deadly Sins became a popular theme among artists in Europe. This helped ingrain them in mass consciousness and culture.

Fortunately, each of the deadly sins has an opposite, corresponding virtue, The Seven Holy Virtues. These are: **Chastity, Abstinence, Liberality, Diligence, Patience, Kindness, and Humility.** Now there's a Progress Challenge if ever there was one!

Go, and sin no more.

The Progress Challenge

Progress in the Balance of Life

Life Is a Smorgasbord

I have had innumerable conversations with a broad range of committed professionals about how they, or others they know, feel overworked and overwhelmed (not to mention underappreciated and underpaid). Solid, proactive folks share with me weekly how they have "no time" to get it all done, and have too many demands placed on them.

> **"There never seems to be enough time to do the things you want to do once you find them."**
> -- *Jim Croce*
> *(For some solid Time Tips, see p.145.)*

Our ideal "stress-free," "healthy," or "right" work-life balance shifts on a daily basis, and certainly over time. The right balance for us tomorrow will probably be different from what it is for us today.

If we want to be working and winning, which includes arriving at that well-worn expression "Healthy Balance," we must begin to internalize our motives, the reasons for our actions. Truly understanding and digging into why we're choosing to do the things we're doing is vital if we're going to reach true balance.

As humans, we have this dangerous and unavailing habit of always looking at the greener grass on the other side of the fence, unaware that it's really all about our priorities and how we roll out our choices, thoughts, and actions.

Progress in the Balance of Life

Working and winning is a unique and personal jigsaw puzzle, and only we can put the pieces together. This puzzle is made up of ourselves, our family, our friends, our work, our career, our interests and hobbies, and, in all of the above, our ideals and aspirations.

I am not saying that comparing ourselves to others is unnatural. I am saying that it is not healthy, productive, or even logical. **All we end up doing is comparing our insides with others' outsides.** We compare the way we feel about our situation as it is today (insides) to the way other people seem to live: career, house, car, family, network – (all "outsides"). This is not fair to either party. We do not know what is going on in the other person's life or head. As my good friend and fellow author Carl Youngberg would say, **"Stop measuring yourself with someone else's yardstick."**

It's like that commercial where the guy has the big house, pool, manicured lawn – the perfect life. He turns to the camera while cruising around his big front yard on his big riding lawn mower and says sadly, *"I am in debt up to my eyeballs."*

Humans love to compete: richer, better-looking, wiser, best-behaved kids, happiest pets, who gets the latest BlackBerry earliest, who understands text-messaging lingo the best. IMHO*, most of this competition is just wasted effort (LOL). Working and winning is a contest with one player – ourselves. The only person we are truly competing against is our current self.

> **"Winning isn't getting ahead of others. It's getting ahead of yourself."**
> --Roger Staubach

* *IMHO = In My Humble Opinion*

Progress in the Balance of Life

Sure, it is natural to compete. None of us wants to look or feel like we're lagging behind. So, if we must compete, let's have our contest be about who smiles (with reason) the most, or who is reaching his or her goals and progressing without stressing. Let's try that. But regardless of their relative merit, and exempting many sports endeavors, most competition appears to be, in essence, foolish, insignificant, absurd, and misguided.

Often, when we are out of *balance*, it is because we're not listening to ourselves. Instead, we're listening to all these other people and their pronouncements about what balance *should* look like. I can't tell you what healthy balance should look like, but I can tell you what it should *feel* like. It should feel like your own nice unique blend of pleasure, peace of mind, profit, pain avoidance, prestige, and power.

One of the main things that gets us out of balance is having too much *stuff*. And I don't mean this just in a physical sense; I also mean in our minds and in our pursuits. It is easy to get scattered, and our world is certainly not trying to help us simplify. For one thing, the sheer volume of information available to us is increasing exponentially. In the 1,500 years between Christ and da Vinci, we had one doubling. Now information doubles every eighteen months.

We must decide and focus on what "in-put" we will put in and act upon – what is most important to us and to the well-being of the people we care about. If we are going to work and win in this world of change, it is vital that we invest the bulk of our time and energy in the activities and goals that offer the highest return on the investment for <u>*our lives*</u>.

Progress in the Balance of Life

We <u>CANNOT</u> do IT ALL or have IT ALL. We can't know everything there is to know or do everything there is to do. We can't watch every movie, eat at every restaurant, travel to every country, or own every electronic gadget. There is no way we can do and have it all. We have to make choices.

> **"Most people struggle with life balance simply because they haven't paid the price to decide what is really important to them."**
> -- *Stephen Covey*

We've all heard the saying, "the trappings of success." *How about the trappings of **excess**?* Our society wants us to want, and needs us to need stuff, but there is a good chance that we don't need or even want a lot of what we already have. *Time for a garage sale?*

Each of us has a mind; we just have to make it up. To progress in the balancing of our lives, we've got to take the hard, uncompromising look inside ourselves to decide what progress means to us. We <u>*can*</u> have and do everything we want *if* we truly ***<u>internalize why</u>*** we want it.

<u>Internalize</u> means to make part of one's own individual thinking and being. <u>Why</u> is the purpose and reasons – meaning the Six Ps of Progress. Passion, desire, and motives for action all come from *internalizing why*. Internalizing takes time, effort, and imagination. We are each unique, with unique lives and unique priorities. There are so many external influences, such as the media, relatives, neighbors, and coworkers, that get in the way of internalizing the whys for our wants. Internalizing helps us become more deliberate in how we choose to react to events, thoughts, images, emotions, etc.

Progress in the Balance of Life

Working and winning comes down to how we roll within ourselves. It is not someone telling us how we *should* invest our time. A balanced life is not *"one-size-fits-all."* Balance in life proceeds from the way we have various options and opportunities sized up in our brain. If we have them positioned and prioritized in a way that helps us *feel* the right mix of the *Six Ps of Progress*, then we are in healthy balance. If we don't, we're not. *Simple, but true.*

It would be so easy if we could read a book wherein the author tells us exactly what a healthy balance is for us, and exactly how we should invest our time.

> **"Step with care and great tact and remember that Life's a Great Balancing Act."**
> -- Dr. Seuss

Do I know how you should invest your time? No.

I don't presume to know how you should invest your time, because I'm not you. I do not know your goals or what progress means to you. I don't even know what you are trying to do or become. *Do you?*

Life is choices.

We must master the choice challenge. We must choose the life we want from all of life's possibilities. If we don't, we run the risk of pursuing goals, buying things, and investing our time the way our boss, significant other, parents, children, neighbors, and advertisers think is best – for them.

Progress in the Balance of Life

We've all heard tales of industrialist dads, pushing their artist children to follow in their footsteps. Certainly what we choose to do should benefit others, but has to mean progress for us, too.

People are attempting to persuade us all the time – to sell us on their ideas – *their* goals for *our* lives! But it's not really a choice of being sold or not being sold. It's simply a choice of whom you are going to be sold by, either yourself or the outside world.

> **"Problems arise in that you have to find a balance between what people need from you and what you need for yourself."**
> *-- Jessye Norman*

It's not that the suggestions that others offer are *"bad"* ways for us to invest our time. A major challenge to progressing in life is that we've got a whole bunch of super-attractive things we can choose to do. For better or worse, life in this age is a smorgasbord, an *all-you-can-live buffet of yummy choices*. Not all the choices on life's smorgasbord are right for us, however, and not all are healthy, or filling.

Imagine you're at a wedding reception. You are about to sit down, and you see a massive buffet table spread out across the back wall of the reception hall. The buffet has everything from roast beef to lobster, from imported Spanish ham to poached salmon, from artichokes to zucchini. You consider getting yourself some grub before you sit down, but some guy at the table says, *"No, no. Sit down. I'll be happy to get you something."* So you sit.

Progress in the Balance of Life

This dude comes back and sets a big plate of food in front of you. You look down and it's got cottage cheese, gray coleslaw, two elderly cherry tomatoes, some kind of green quiche-looking thing, runny red Jell-O, and about half a pound of pickled okra. Talk about an unbalanced plate. You think, *"I don't want any of this stuff! I wanted some of the prime rib and smoked salmon!"*

So, now you have some choices. You may:
- A. Eat or pick disgustedly at what has been selected for you.
- B. Sit there and go hungry.
- C. Get up and fix your own plate.

If we don't choose, we lose. So much of what is out there in the world is irrelevant to what we want to achieve in our lives. Unless we have a true concept of who we are and what we want from the smorgasbord of life, someone will be only too happy to fix a plate for us. And the plate they fix will consist of what they want us to have based on their own reasons, their whys. We're the only ones who can fix our plate our way.

> **"You gotta fight, fight, fight for your mind, while you got the time."**
> *-- Ben Harper*

Each of us has the need and the power, and hears the personal imperative, to craft our own goals and to utilize our resources (time, money, networks, knowledge) to make them happen.

Life is a smorgasbord, so fix yourself a balanced plate – and dig in!

Ponder & Progress: A Life in the Balance

1. What does life balance mean to you?

2. When do you feel out of balance?

3. What do you want from the smorgasbord of life?

4. What's lacking in your life right now? Why?

5. What is there too much of? Why?

6. When do you feel that you are working and winning?

7. Do you need to simplify? What's stopping you?

8. Is comparing yourself to others resulting in your feeling out of balance? When? Why?

9. How should you invest your time?

10. What will bring you the right mix of the Six Ps of Progress?

"Life is like riding a bicycle.
To keep your balance you must keep moving."
-- Albert Einstein

Too Stressed to Progress

"When I hear somebody sigh, 'Life is hard,'
I am always tempted to ask, 'compared to what?'"
-- *Sydney Harris*

Over the years I've been surprised by the number of professionals in my boot camps and in one-on-one coaching who have shared with me their sense of being overwhelmed, underappreciated, and underpaid. Workplace stress is rarely part of anyone's job description, but it is unfortunately part of most jobs. It is tough to progress when we are stressed. In fact, we *feel* stress when we *feel* we are being *hindered from progressing*.

How to deal with or relate to the stressful stimuli in this high-tech, low-touch world of speed-of-light change is a vital and important topic that desperately needs discussion.

Check this: **Stress not only limits your progress; stress can and will kill you (if you don't take action)!**
- The American Medical Association says that stress is now the basic cause of over 60% of all diseases and illnesses (cancer, heart problems, etc.).
- Stress-related problems, according to the American Institute for Stress, are responsible for 75 % to 90 % of doctor visits.
- A study conducted by the University of London found that *unmanaged reactions* to stress were more likely to lead to cancer and heart disease than either smoking cigarettes or eating foods high in the bad kind of cholesterol.

Progress in the Balance of Life – Stress

Virtually no part of the body escapes the ravages of prolonged negative stress. Unfortunately, many of us make up our minds to "get serious" about our physical and mental health only when we become ill, suffer a heart attack, or experience some other form of breakdown.

Stress is very dangerous, not to mention expensive. Businesses across the U.S. of A. lose $200-$300 billion dollars annually to stress, resulting in loss in productivity (i.e., less progress) and treatment costs. Effects of stress in the workplace include absenteeism, disruptive outbursts, and the tendency to do as little as possible to get by.
All reduce productivity and damage an organization's bottom line. Plus, many of us do not have a well-defined boundary between work and home, and end up taking work problems home with us and letting them affect our personal life.

> **"If you are distressed by anything external, the pain is not due to the thing itself, but to your estimate of it; and this you have the power to revoke at any moment."**
> *-- Marcus Aurelius*

I don't mean to stress you out about stress, but the crazy thing to consider is that WE are truly the ultimate *cause* of our own stress. It is our reaction to stressful stimuli that "makes us sick," not the stimuli themselves. We internalize too much outside pressure, which causes inside pressures. No matter what the circumstance, we still have power over the attitude we take toward it. When we feel stress, we become focused on the pain and not the opportunities to take positive steps.

> **Often, we invest so much time dealing with stress that we don't take time to progress.**

Progress in the Balance of Life – Stress

We all relate to stimuli differently. What really freaks one person out may excite another, or only mildly irritate a third person. The key is to know in advance positive ways to respond to stressful stimuli.

When our negative reactions to the little stuff build up, it undermines our ability to progress. We become irritable and worn out, which leads to more stress. This is an inappropriate triggering of a very useful survival mechanism. When we're in fight-or-flight mode, we NEED to focus on negatives *(no time to smell the flowers when we're running from a burning building)*. But when the same physiological reaction is in response to social situations, we only see the negatives, and lose sight of our strengths and resources.

We often think of stressful stimuli as the big life stuff – like a challenging relationship or a scary economic climate. But a great deal of our anxiety comes from the little day-to-day pressures commonly faced in today's workplace. This dear old world is full of possible "stressors":
- Dissatisfied customers and indecisive prospects
- Our kids, our coworkers, our coworkers' kids
- Technology challenges and industry shifts
- Unrealistic workloads and deadlines
- Slow computers, slow microwaves
- Office gossip and competition
- Long unorganized meetings
- Long commutes in traffic
- Disorganized work area
- Dictatorial leadership
- Cell phones & spam
- Physical ailments

These are but a few of the world's never-ending supply of stimuli that we may choose to freak out over, or calmly face.

Progress in the Balance of Life – Stress

Our power lies in never losing sight of the fact that it's our <u>choice</u> to get stressed by something or not get stressed by something. We have the choice to be happy, to be mad, to be stressed, to be giddy. *I like giddy.* Nothing can MAKE us stressed, just like, despite the suggestion of many a love song, we can't MAKE someone happy, or vice versa. We can do things we think will encourage them to choose to be happy, but we can not MAKE someone happy. It is their choice. To be stressed is ours. When we are stressed, we are choosing to respond to stimuli in a stressful way. Stress may be normal, but is not necessary.

You control you.
You only control you.
Only you control you.
You control you only.

It feels great to give 110% at work, but it's important to always remember that taking good care of ourselves pays off professionally as well as emotionally. Develop stress immunity and resilience. Invest time in doing what helps you renew your energy. If we are going to put ourselves in the best possible position to work and win in this world of change, it is vital that we take back control of our lives and careers by *choosing* to gain control of our thought processes. Pretending that the stress stimuli are not all around us only increases the problem. The way to progress is through recognition and action.

> **"When we commit to action, to actually doing something rather than feeling trapped by events, the stress in our life becomes manageable."**
> *-- Greg Anderson*

Ponder & Progress: Too Stressed to Progress

1. When do you feel overworked and overwhelmed?

2. What are you allowing yourself to get stressed about?

3. What physical challenges are you having that may be related to stress?

4. Do you have trouble sleeping due to stress?

5. Is it time to get serious about your stress?

6. How can you be better prepared for stressful stimuli?

7. How can you choose *not* to stress?

8. Do you have too many demands on your time?

9. Are you too stressed to progress?

10. Can you DO something about a stressful situation? Bet you CAN, and if you can …DO IT.

> "Stress is the trash of modern life – we all generate it but if you don't dispose of it properly, it will pile up and overtake your life."
> -- Danzae Pace

From Stress to Progress: Ten Tips

1. Make Some YOU Time.
YOU time is not a luxury. YOU time is not wasted time. We all need to turn it down a bit from time to time. YOU time is vital to your progress. Invest time in relaxing. The key is the mental break. Don't even think about feeling guilty about this YOU time. Fun and leisure are vital for recharging our lives.

- Read a book or magazine *(the one you just haven't had time to read)*.
- Watch your favorite childhood movie.
- Have coffee with a friend.
- Visit a museum or library.
- Take a power nap.
- Listen to your soothing, relaxing music.
- Get a hobby.
- Stretch.
- Meditate.
- Garden.
- Take a hot shower or warm bath.
- Get a massage. *Maybe you have the need to be kneaded.*
- Take a vacation; even a 20-minute one can help.

Important Note: Vacations should be vacations. It's not a vacation if you're reading business emails and taking a bunch of business calls. Set boundaries between work and the rest of your life. If we can't completely detach from work, we are unable to receive the benefits of the attempted rest.

When and how do you relax?

Progress in the Balance of Life – Stress

2. Think Lovely Thoughts.*
Yes, I am talking about affirmations. We use affirmations all the time; it's just that most of them are negative, stress-inducing, and self-limiting.
>"My job stinks."
>"I am stressed out."
>"I can't catch a break."

Our brains are trippy and complicated, and can do amazing things. But at their core, our brains want one thing:
To Be Right. Whatever we continually tell ourselves about ourselves and our lives, our brains are working overtime to make true. Visualize the good. Practice self-talk that emphasizes a self-affirming attitude.
Stuff like:
>"I can handle this."
>"I make good decisions."
>"I am having a good day."

It is imperative that we be careful about the things we say to ourselves, and to talk to ourselves as a winner to a winner. As I mentioned earlier, *your brain is a terrible thing to use against yourself.*

***Think Lovely Thoughts** is what Peter Pan told John, Michael, and Wendy they would have to do to learn to fly in the song, "I'm Flying." Peter also blew fairy dust on them but I don't know where you can get your hands on any of that. The kids came up with lovely thoughts like: Fishing, Hoopskirt, Candy, Picnics, Summer, More Candy, Sailing, Flowers, still more Candy, and Christmas.*

What are lovely thoughts to you?

Progress in the Balance of Life – Stress

3. Say YES to NO.
Most of us take on too many responsibilities, try to do too much, and even own too much. Being too busy is a big source of stress in today's *get, get, get and go, go, go* world. Often, we are so chronically over-scheduled that we never give ourselves a chance to offer our best or to enjoy the moment.

Are your days fulfilling, or are they merely full?
It is possible that we could get more out of life by doing less. When we internalize the difference between *full* and *fulfilling*, we realize it's not how many events we attend, activities we get involved in, or how much stuff we have that's important. We do not have to say "yes" to every demand on OUR time. And we shouldn't feel bad, since we are saying "no" to the event or project, not the person.

Being busy can wear us out. If we are committed to working and winning in this world of change, we must know our limits and not limit our NOs.
- Consider your well-crafted goals and your schedule before agreeing to additional work.
- Simplify – get rid of the clutter and baggage in your life and in your house. Say NO to clutter.
- Start your own *Just Say NO* campaign to regain quality time. Review priorities and see if a request fits. When you see things that waste time or hinder your progress, speak up.
- Stop trying to make everyone happy. (We can't do it anyway.)

A polite way to say NO to a request for YOUR time:
"I'm quite committed. I can be your backup, but please keep searching."
[Find more insight on "Time Management" on p. 145]

Progress in the Balance of Life – Stress

4. Air In. Air Out.
Deep breathing is one of the best stress-relief methods, often recommended but rarely utilized. Deep breathing works as long as you don't do it right in front of your boss or a customer. Here is the classic method in a four-step process:
Step 1: *Close your eyes and focus only on breathing.**
Step 2: *Take in a slow <u>deep</u> breath.*
Step 3: *Hold for three to five seconds.*
Step 4: *Slowly exhale.*
Repeat five to 10 times, as needed. Whether you breathe in through the nose and/or out through the mouth, is irrelevant. It is the deep abdominal breathing that's inherently relaxing.
*Do keep eyes open if driving or playing racquetball.

5. Find and Create Humor.
As legendary director Mel Brooks said, *"Humor is just another defense against the universe."* Our minds can only focus on one thing at a time. When we find the humor in a situation, it automatically relieves stress because the humor takes the place of stress, washing it away in waves of laughter and sometimes even rivers of tears. Laughter is good medicine.

Humor is a learned coping skill that improves with practice. When we laugh, similar to when we exercise, endorphins are released in the brain that help us feel better about the situation and offer more energy to tackle challenges. "Belly laughs" are also said to give our innards a good workout, massaging our organs while warming our hearts. *Touching, isn't it?*

> **"A person without a sense of humor is like a wagon without springs – jolted by every pebble on the road."**
> *-- Henry Ward Beecher*

Humor also happens to be profitable. People are drawn to people who are upbeat and have a positive, jovial frame of mind. Professionals who maintain a sense of humor gain respect. Find what makes you laugh. And be sure to laugh at yourself from time to time.

What makes you laugh?
Where is the humor in the situation?

6. Break a Sweat and Let Off Some Steam.
Have you heard about this new craze? They call it...regular exercise! When our lives seem to be up in the air, exercise can keep us grounded. Exercise releases mood-enhancing, feel-good chemicals like endorphins, the mind-body's natural painkiller and mood-calmer. We feel better when we get a good workout in. Plus, exercise gives us a positive sense of accomplishment – and our clothes don't fit as tightly.

It is recommended that we shoot for 30 minutes of some good sweaty physical activity three to four times a week. But even five minutes here and there throughout the day is going to make a difference in how we view stressful stimuli.

Even brisk walking and light stretching feel good and can help you stay in control. Be your own bouncer and take it outside. Fresh air and natural full-spectrum light add checks to the *Good for You* column. The main thing is to find ways of exercising that are fun for you.

Find exercise lonely or boring?
Get a friend to break a sweat with you. I bet they could use the exercise and the endorphins just as much as you.

Progress in the Balance of Life – Stress

7. Budget Your Spending, and Save, Save, Save.
We all know that debt is a big, big problem. Statistics on American household debt are astounding. Living in the shadow of mountainous debt leaves little room for light or air. Its presence, always lumbering overhead and ever on our mind, means constant stress. And if we should momentarily forget about it, the phone is sure to ring at dinnertime with a friendly reminder from the Bank of Interruptions.

To meet the progress challenge, we must be willing to alter our spending behavior so we can sleep nights and get to where we want to be.
- Establish financial goals. ***Commit*** to achieving them.
- Pay off your whole credit card bill each month.
- Don't wait to start saving. Time is ticking.
- Get enough life insurance.
- Do not let emotions drive buying or investment decisions.

All of the above help us go from stress to progress.

8. Sleep tight and right.
A fresh mind and body are better able to relate powerfully to stressful stimuli. Let there be no doubt: Our minds and bodies need down-time for rejuvenation. Get seven to eight hours of sleep every night. *Yeah, I know – seven to eight every night is tough.* At least go to bed at the same time each night. Give your mind and body the rest they need to recharge.

It is common when we are stressed to have difficulty in falling asleep, even if we have made it to bed at a good hour. This really stinks, because the stress has already worn us out and now we can't nod off, which makes us even more stressed, tired, irritable, and unable to progress.

Progress in the Balance of Life – Stress

When having trouble falling asleep, take a warm shower or bath and try not to focus on the effects of *not* sleeping because that will just keep you from sleeping.

You might even consider trying Viktor Frankl's technique of paradoxical intent. That is, if all else fails, pretend that you must stay awake, or convince yourself that staying awake is a good thing, that nothing bad will come of it, and that it will give you a great opportunity to let your mind wander. Putting a jolly spin on sleeplessness, even if it at first feels phony, will at least calm you down, and may even work in the way that Frankl envisioned.

9. Give Mind and Body the "Right Fuel."

Challenges take energy. A lack of the "right fuel" can cause a bunch of problems like fatigue, lack of concentration, low morale, halitosis, death-by-Twinkies, etc. Our minds and bodies respond more effectively to stressful stimuli when they are getting the right nutrients. Give your body the right fuel for life's challenges.

> "Tell me what you eat,
> I'll tell you who you are."
> -- Anthelme Brillat-Savarin

Hey, I'm not the guru on nutrition, and you don't need one anyway. You know what the "Right Fuel" is. It's the stuff we try to make kids eat.

As for drinking alcohol:
Hangovers never add to the bottom line.

Progress in the Balance of Life – Stress

10. Become Flexible in Problem Solving.
Allow yourself the time to work through challenges and find the best, possibly new or unique, way to progress. Be willing to try new solutions. Long commutes and driving in heavy traffic can seem like a big waste of time. Use that time to progress. Have mind-expanding CDs to listen to. Rigid thinking encourages stress.
- Don't let assumptions limit possible solutions.
- Chop up big problems and challenges into smaller ones. Address each component individually.
- Ask several people for their advice and suggestions.
- Alter your point of view. Imagine yourself as a child, a billionaire, or even riding on a beam of light.

How would you view the challenge from this new perspective?

<u>Important Note:</u>
If you feel like your stress is just too much, talk with your family, a friend, or a counselor. Ask for help. Talk it out. Do not let stress impede your progress. ***The strong get help.***

Be Progress.

<u>Beam me up, Einstein</u>
It is said that Albert Einstein imagined riding on a beam of light when he came up with his theory of relativity.
Pretty good theory.

Always Time to Progress

Time is the great equalizer. Each day, every one of us gets the same amount – 24 hours – 1440 minutes. Nobody gets less. Nobody gets more. Time can not be slowed, stopped, sped up, or saved like money. Time's ticking, always ticking.

What is an effective use of your time?
The answer is totally subjective because the value of the results is subjective. What makes a wise investment of time for me may not be a wise investment for you. Each of us is, however, investing some of our time in daily activities that do not serve our goals. Too much time is allotted to fleeting interests that we know are less important than progressing toward our crafted goals. That is why it is so important to remind ourselves of the benefits of our goals.

> **"You only live once, but if you do it right, once is enough."**
> *-- Mae West*

All of us have said to ourselves, *"Oh, I really would like to (fill in the blank), if I could only FIND the time."* Time does not need to be *found*. It is right here. Time needs to be invested wisely. Each day we are *choosing* to invest our time somewhere, and for a reason. By managing our time more wisely, we minimize stress, improve our quality of life, and have time to *progress*. Unfortunately, time management is one of those life skills that no one teaches us in school.

**Time Management is really
Self-Management, with a respect for time.**

Ponder & Progress: Always Time to Progress

1. *When do you feel you waste time?*

2. *Is procrastination a problem? How so?*

3. *Do you need to exercise better "time management?" Why?*

4. *What are two important things in your life that must be done but aren't?*

5. *What are the most valuable uses of your time right now?*

6. *Do you list and rank tasks that need to be done each day?*

7. *During what part of the day are you most productive or effective?*

8. *What are two actions that you do weekly that could and should be done by someone else?*

9. *What is the best use of your time in terms of your short-term goals?*

10. *What is the best use of your time in terms of your long-term goals?*

> **"I am definitely going to take a course on time management…just as soon as I can work it into my schedule."**
> -- Louis E. Boone

Progress in the Balance of Life – Time

Always Time to Progress: Ten Tips

1. "To Do" or Not "To Do"
In the late 1920s, Charles Schwab, president of the then fledgling Bethlehem Steel Company (unrelated to the discount brokerage of the same name), asked management consultant and efficiency expert Ivy Lee to help him and his team become more productive. After observing Schwab for several hours, Ivy told him that he could teach a time-management system in about 20 minutes that would enable Schwab and his executives to get 50% more work done, without working harder or longer. Schwab asked what this advice would cost him. Lee replied, *"Use the plan for six months and send me a check for how much you think it is worth."*

Lee recommended the following:
1. Write down the things you have to do the following day.
2. Number these tasks in the order of their real importance.
3. Start your day by working on the first item on your list and stick with it until it's accomplished (or until you've done as much as you can); then go on to the next one, and so on.

Six months later, Lee received a check from Schwab for $25,000, equivalent to $400,000 in today's world.
Four hundred thousand dollars – for a To-Do List tip?
I should have charged more for this book!

Charles Schwab and his executives took Ivy's "To-Do List" advice, and within five years turned Bethlehem Steel Company into the biggest steel producer in the world.

A To-Do List is common sense, right? But is it common practice?

The key is to address the most important thing first, and not to look over the additional fifteen "To-Do" items until Number One is completed. That way, we won't see Number Twelve and say, *"Oh, that won't take very long, so I'll do that first. It's easier."* Prioritizing ensures that we are investing our time and energy in those tasks and steps that bring the biggest benefits to our lives. *If we don't know what we should be doing, how can we manage our time to do it?*

> **"If you want to make good use of your time, you've got to know what's most important and then give it all you've got."**
> -- Lee Iacocca

It is OK, and normal, to have stuff left on your list at the end of the day. If you follow Ivy's system, you have worked on the most important thing already. The other stuff flows through to the next day.

Daren Martin, my good friend, told me that when he gets to work, he devotes at least an hour to the most important thing on his To-Do List even before he checks his email. He says that even if he can't get this most important thing done in an hour or so, he's likely to get back to it quickly because he has gotten it going. Go, Daren.

Some folks feel compelled to write out their To-Do List by hand, saying they feel it instills more commitment into each item because they are willing to rewrite it each day until the item gets crossed off. There's also the thought that the act of physically writing on paper somehow sets the task in cerebral-stone, making it more likely to be accomplished. *Cool. Rock on.*

Progress in the Balance of Life – Time

Other folks prefer to use some form of time-management software that can break their list into manageable chunks. *Again, cool. Rock on.*

Figure out what works for you and don't "make a big to-do" (old idiom for "complain too much") about it. Just do the "To Do."

2. Construct Structure by Planning with a Planner.
Most successful Progress Agents have some kind of time-management system – BlackBerry, paper day planner, *something*. Keep it with you at all times, adding to it and striking off completed items, and set aside time for specific tasks like prospecting, networking, and follow-ups. Setting a specific time period – even a specific place – to make calls significantly increases the chances of actually doing it. Reduce the risk of procrastination, time-frittering, and "puttering" by formalizing tasks.

> **We don't find time or make it;
> we schedule time and take it.**

When using a planner, be sure to track your goals and your use of time. Solid tracking helps develop a better sense of what we can accomplish in a given period of time.

3. Set a Realistic Schedule.
It is common to overestimate how much can be done within a given time and try to pack too much into our day. The residues of a crowded day are often frustration, careless errors, disappointment, and even self-punishment. And it is not just we who suffer. The people in our day suffer as well because we are scattered, stressed, unprepared, and late for appointments. When traveling, be sure to factor in time for

Progress in the Balance of Life – Time

gridlock and other delays, so you're in the state you need to be in when you arrive at where you need to be.

Setting realistic schedules gives us a little time to chill. Chilling doesn't mean turning off. Giving ourselves a little breathing room enables us to think things through, regroup, refocus, or maybe come up with new ideas that could positively impact our business life.

4. Delegate Right.
We can accomplish a lot more with help. We shouldn't just delegate to full-time employees. Delegating can also include others whom we turn to so that we can progress in other ways. Outsourcing is delegating. I outsource my lawn care, bookkeeping, and pizza baking. (Thanks, Pizza Hut.)

Delegation is not dumping. As leaders, if something we assign doesn't get done right, it is on us. Either WE:
- A.) did not communicate the task clearly enough, and/or provide the right tools; or we
- B.) delegated the task to the <u>wrong</u> person.

Delegating to *wrong* person with *wrong* info leads to change.
Delegating to *right* person with *wrong* info leads to change.
Delegating to *wrong* person with *right* info leads to change.
Delegating to *right* person with *right* info leads to **<u>progress.</u>**
The right info means providing:
- Clear goals (Objectives must be clear, but allow attendant procedures to vary. Guard against any tendency you may have to micro-manage.)
- Training (classroom and/or on the job)
- Realistic deadlines (Make sure those you delegate to know the relative importance of the task.)
- Rewards/Consequences

Progress in the Balance of Life – Time

What on your To-Do List can be handled by someone else? What are some things you are doing daily that others could do, so that you would have the time to do the things YOU want to do?

> "In truth, people can generally make time for what they choose to do; it is not really the time but the will that is lacking."
> -- Sir John Lubbock

5. Focus on Being Effective More Than Being Efficient.
There's a big difference between "effectiveness" and "efficiency." When we are efficient, we are able to carry out tasks in a short time. However, we won't be effective unless those actions result in us moving closer to our goals.

<u>Efficiency</u> basically means producing outcomes quickly. <u>Effectiveness</u> basically means producing desired outcomes.

Sometimes, becoming more efficient leads to becoming less effective. For example, in this fast pace of life and business, we naturally seek more efficient ways to communicate. We send e-mails rather than make phone calls, and have phone meetings rather than meeting face-to-face. Although these may appear to be more efficient ways to communicate, they may actually be less effective than the methods they replace.

Clearly, being both effective and efficient should be the aim, but if effectiveness is lost for the sake of efficiency, then the whole purpose for doing whatever it is we're doing is defeated. Sales calls can be made very efficiently, twenty-five an hour. But if sales or appointments are the goal, the calls are not very effective. We can deal with customer issues efficiently, but not necessarily effectively.

Sometimes we are simply doing the wrong things. In his book, *The 4-Hour Workweek,* Timothy Ferriss shares how we shouldn't waste time being efficient in tasks that are not effective, and that we should work to limit or eliminate such time-wasters.

The 80-20 Rule, or Pareto Principle, states that 80 percent of the reward or effect from any endeavor comes from 20 percent of the effort. The trick to being effective is to isolate and identify that valuable 20 percent and put most of your energy into those efforts.

There is definitely a need for efficiency. But efficiency is never the goal. Effectiveness is what is ultimately important, and effectiveness is personal. Nothing vital should be given up for the sake of being efficient. Better to do the right thing wrong, than the wrong thing right. Of course, it is best to do the right things right. **Working and winning is mastering ways to efficiently be more effective at "being progress."**

80+20 words on the Pareto Principle
Twentieth-century management consultant Joseph M. Juran coined this well-established principle, naming it after Italian economist and philosopher Vilfredo Pareto. Pareto had observed that 80% of his country's wealth was controlled by 20% of its population. Juran, whose teachings focused on managing for quality, expanded Pareto's principle, applying it to productivity issues. (For example, 80% of our sales come from 20% of our customers.) Although the principle is also known as "the vital few and the trivial many," Joseph Juran preferred "the vital few and the useful many" as a way to show that the remaining 80% should not be ignored.

Progress in the Balance of Life – Time

6. Create Progress Blocks.
Block out time for important tasks, such as making calls, reading trades, opening mail, taking a nap. (I am not kidding.) Blocking time is especially useful when dealing with email. Just because someone can contact us immediately via email doesn't mean that we must reply immediately. Most people are not looking for an immediate response, just a timely one.

I used to check email every time I'd hear the *Bing!* "You've got mail." Now I turn off the sound. It's simply not an effective investment of time to read and answer each and every email as it arrives. As long as our most important contacts know how to reach us in an emergency, we can schedule email correspondence for four to six times per day.

7. Make a Molehill Out of the Mountain.
JOKE -   Q: How do you eat an elephant?
          A: One bite at a time.
Most of the time, starting projects is more challenging than finishing them. We see this big project we'd love to accomplish, we doubt we will ever finish it, so we don't even start. The key to *putting off putting off* is to break projects into manageable chunks, so we are not overwhelmed by them. Start!

> "He who has begun has half done.
> Dare to be wise; begin!"
> -- *Horace*

8. Build More Priceless Business Relationships.
Is this a time-management tip? You bet. The more priceless business relationships we have, the quicker and more efficiently we can get things done. Get out there and crack the networking CODE.

9. Dare to Take Time.
If we don't have the time to do it right, we don't have time to do it wrong. Doing our work right the first time often takes more time upfront, but correcting a flurry of careless errors usually results in more time spent in the long run. I know it may sound odd, but often good time management means responding slower to some tasks.

For example, if we are investing time in a high-priority activity, we might not answer the phone while we're doing it. We need to take the time we need to do a quality job.

> "Until we manage time, we can manage nothing else."
> -- Peter Drucker

10. Know Your Progress Clock.
Try to schedule important activities and tough projects during your period of peak productivity. *When is that?* Everybody is different, but each of us has a time of day (or night) when we tend to be most productive.

To figure out yours, try keeping a *Take Time for Progress* journal for one or two weeks. Record tasks performed and associated time values to uncover time that can be utilized more wisely. Identify time-wasters. We can learn a great deal by monitoring ourselves at 30-minute intervals. At every half hour, consider: *What behaviors must be altered to progress?* Design your daily schedule to keep your best time available for YOUR most important projects.

There is Always Time to Progress.

Be Progress.

The Progress Challenge

Finding Progress in Change

Stop, BOP, & Roll
Finding Progress in Change

Every day, every hour, every minute, we're changing and so is our world. Some may feel resistant to change, and even claim to be personally unchangeable, yet the presence of change is one of the few constants. Marriage, graduation, a new job, the birth of a child: all bring change. But so do eating a big lunch, seeing a sad movie, and meeting someone new. We experience and relate to change daily. Every day we have a slightly new normal.

Significant change can arrive like an Oklahoma twister, picking us up, shaking our sense of identity, and then dropping us way outside of our comfort zone. The ailing economy and the tough business climate (not to mention the real climate) make it easy to understand why so many people have trouble finding ways to get and stay moving toward progress. Yet, opportunities for progress still exist, even in the most challenging of times.

Working and winning in a world of change requires new processes, heightened performance, and traveling untrodden paths. It is tough and more than a tad scary to let go of the familiar and the sense of security that familiarity provides. We often want to skip the period of transition and quickly get to the other side in order to regain some level of comfort. When dealing with uncertainty, we should be careful not to move too quickly and miss the opportunity to move forward.

Here are the three keys to staying confident and productive through the necessary process of finding progress in change. **Stop, BOP, and Roll** your way to progress.

Stop

Stop Beating Yourself (and Others) Up.
We are not perfect – *and wouldn't we feel out of place if we were?* Many of us harbor perfectionist standards for ourselves (as well as for others) that are simply unhealthy and unrealistic. *Not good.*

> "Never discourage anyone...who continually makes progress, no matter how slow."
> -- *Plato* (That "anyone" includes you!)

When we focus on beating ourselves up, we are tearing down our level of resolve and persistence. Believe me, there are plenty of people out there who are only too willing to do that for us. Cut yourself (and others) some slack. <u>We do not have to be perfect to Be Progress.</u>

Stop Blaming Others and Holding on to the Past.
It is natural to have difficulty accepting and adjusting to change and uncertainty, especially changes we didn't initiate or think we wanted. Put issues into perspective by focusing on the big picture. Don't focus on the injustice. Focus on your next proactive step.

If we are not careful, we can waste an enormous amount of quality time and energy dwelling on, resenting, and second-guessing the actions of others. This type of thinking can stifle our creativity and our imagination. We get stuck. It is weird to consider, but we can even get comfortable being stuck, because shifting our thoughts is often perceived as being more painful.

Finding Progress in Change

It helps to begin recognizing the events that don't truly have much effect on our lives and letting them go without getting down on ourselves about letting them go. I am not saying that events don't have consequences, but letting stress and self-doubt impede our progress does not have to be one of them. Things have changed before. Things have progressed before. The only past we should hold onto are the reminders of *past progress*.

Where is your next step forward?
Believe you should take it and take it. Don't doubt yourself. Make something good happen.

Stop Procrastinating!
It doesn't matter how skilled we are or how determined we say we are if procrastination keeps us from getting rolling. Here are the ABC's of why we procrastinate.

A. **We are not truly 100% committed.**
We really can't say, *"I am committed; I just haven't done anything yet."* When we're truly committed – WE ACT.

B. **We fear failure.**
Ralph Waldo Emerson knew the way around this universal challenge, but most of all he knew the way *through* it: *"Do the thing you fear, and the death of fear is certain."* Action helps remove fear and doubt.

C. **We don't know enough to do the task**.
If we don't know how to do something, we have to find out. There are countless ways (books, programs, co-workers, clergy, the Internet) to find reliable info on solid next steps.

Finding Progress in Change

Stop Letting Feelings of the Moment get in the Way.
There is often a big gap between what we *want* to do and what we *feel* like doing. What we want to do is based on anticipated consequences and educated guesses as to what feelings will be reached. What we *feel* like doing is based on how we *feel* at the moment (tricky). Here is the real kicker: We work best when these are aligned.

Muhammad Ali, arguably the greatest boxer who ever lived, is quoted as saying, *"I hated every minute of the training, but I said, 'Don't quit. Suffer now and live the rest of your life as a champion.'"* He didn't say he didn't *want* to train. He said he *hated* to train. He trained despite his feelings about training. He wanted to train because of the benefits of the results he would achieve. He *wanted* to do something he didn't feel like doing because of the progress he would feel. He didn't feel like training but he trained anyway because of outcomes he looked forward to in the future. We mustn't let what we feel like doing hold us back from our progress.

Sometimes we're going to have to vacuum the house, make the outbound calls, pump the iron, skip the desserts, set the alarm, or numerous other acts of will that are not super fun in the moment. But feelings can change quickly. It is vital to base our actions on feelings we aspire to enjoy in the future, and not only on what we feel like doing in a particular moment *(tough to do, but essential)*.

> **"Life has a habit of not standing hitched. You got to ride it like you find it."**
> *-- Woody Guthrie*

Stop Changing and Start Progressing.
I've already covered this. *Moving on.*

Finding Progress in Change

BOP – Be Open to Progress

It may be uncomfortable and even painful, but we must *shift our focus to the possible* if we are to harness our potential and make progress. Each of us has unbelievable potential, which, for the most part, is only limited by our minds. Our mind-set is the first thing we have to empower if we're going to find progress in change.

This is especially true in this ever-changing, always challenging marketplace. While any number of actions and initiatives may be employed to progress, our minds must first be willing. When the going gets tough, the mind has to get tough to get going.

It takes guts to confront an uncertain future. But that future, though unpredictable, also brings the possibility of progress. Even unwanted "change" can present opportunities, but we've got to be in the right mental state to identify and pounce on them. Turbulence and problems are life forces that may be seen as opportunities for growth and advancement. As Albert Einstein said, *"In the middle of difficulty lies opportunity."*

Be open to change as an opportunity to progress. Acceptance evokes our personal power to navigate change and create progress. Some transitions are welcomed and some are not. Either way, recognize that we are engaged in a transition, and our attention is needed.

> **"When you're finished changing, you're finished."**
> *-- Benjamin Franklin*

Finding Progress in Change

We create our future with our responses to change. Interact with the change, get intimate with it. In bop music of the 1940s, musical interaction between the soloist and the drummer was referred to as "dropping bombs." We cannot control what happens to us, but we can control our reaction to what happens to us. When the world "drops bombs" and sends its jazzy licks our way, we need to feel we have bombs to drop as well that will put us back in the groove (or at least know where we can find shelter).

Be ready, willing, and able to improvise. When we open up to new experiences, we discover potential in ourselves we never knew we had. Often, it takes more effort not to do something than to do it. It helps to be flexible in how we view problems. We need to quit burning up our energy in shooting down ideas. Latch on to a couple of ideas and go for it. Think *"I'll do it"* instead of *"Not me,"* or *"This won't work."*

Invent your future by committing to lifelong learning. Knowing that change is coming and even why we must change is not enough; it helps to know how to progress. Be ready for the world and its endless opportunities for progress. Learn what you need to learn, and more.

Action steps often need time to work. It's important to give them that time. However, we must also be open-minded enough to know when to use alternate approaches and strategies to move forward. Commit to progress, not to a plan. Commit to action. Keep your eyes, ears, mind, and heart open for ways to progress.

Be Open to Progress.

Finding Progress in Change

Dropping Bombs on Bop
World War II played a big role in bringing about bop music. The war after "The War to End All Wars" drafted many of the established musicians of the day to play in the armed forces' big bands. Younger musicians, like Dizzy Gillespie, Charlie Parker, and Thelonious Monk (many teenagers, and too young to be drafted), were left to play in clubs and touring bands.

Financial cutbacks and an entertainment tax (both brought on by the war effort) encouraged these young musicians to make do with less. In streamlining their bands to four to six musicians, they'd unwittingly created a perfect vehicle for exploring the improvisational elements of jazz and blues music.

Freed from the demands and constraints of the Big Band arrangements, these smaller bebop groups allowed for a flowing improvisation among all the musicians. Bop became a new direction for jazz, and a new art form unto itself.

Rhythmically in bop music, the steady beat is assigned to the bass player and the ride and hi-hat cymbals of the drummer. This new approach allowed drummers (like Max Roach) to interact with the soloist, creating rhythmic accents with the bass drum and snare, almost like a shifting call and response. This interaction in bop music was referred to as "dropping bombs."

Jamming musically is not so different from improvisation with, and attunement to, the situations and people we interact with every day. All of us can BOP our way to progressive rhythms in our own lives.

Finding Progress in Change

Roll

Make action the way you roll. As Will Rogers said, *"Even if you are on the right track, you'll get run over if you just sit there."* Consistently be doing something you believe will help you move toward progress.

Start now. Take some action. Be dynamic. Dare to fail. Time is ticking. The sooner you find out what doesn't work, the sooner you will find out what will. And the sooner you start, the sooner you will progress. With each small step you grow in confidence. The excitement level increases.

Think of some action that you could take that you believe would help you advance by even a baby-step toward your goal. Take that step. Progress is one-step-at-a-time forward. Take today's step. Give it your best shot. Take risks. *Try, you never know...*

> *"...sometimes they go in."*
> -- *Jerry Dean Lindsay Sr.*
> *(Avid golfer and rabid optimist. Rest in Peace, Far Far.)*

Focus on NOW rather than Later. Today is all we have, so make the most of it. *Got a new idea, a way to tweak an existing sales practice, customer-service initiatives, or a step you could take toward your goals?* The best time to do anything about it is N-O-W.

Focus on what you are doing today to move you or your company toward the goal, rather than thinking, *"I have to wait for this thing or that thing to happen first."* <u>There will always be a reason for not taking action.</u>

Finding Progress in Change

Procrastinators can find every reason under the sun. Don't wait for that one big thing to happen before you move forward. And don't wait for the right mood to strike. Do one small thing today that you believe will help you find progress in change, no matter how small. The point is to start immediately. Stop reading this and go do it – *but then please come back!*

Develop the *Do it now* habit. Be assertive. Be proactive. You are most likely on a learning curve, so round that corner. After assessing the likely consequences, make it okay to fail, to try new things. It's how we grow, wise up, progress. *Haven't we heard all this before?*

The Progress Agent's Two Step System for Progress

Step 1: Get Reliable Information.
Step 2: Act on Reliable Information.

That's it – two steps, simple. Get reliable information and act on reliable information. If the information turns out not to be useful, *guess what we do?* Get reliable information and act on reliable information, over and over and over and over.

> "When any real progress is made, we unlearn and learn anew what we thought we knew before."
> -- Henry David Thoreau

Today, information is readily available for the asking. Good info is everywhere – on the Internet, in books, recordings, and seminars. Really, not knowing how to do something is the weakest of excuses.

Finding Progress in Change

If we want something badly enough, there are ways to get the info we need, even if we have to pay someone for it. Instead of thinking, *I don't know how,* ask yourself, *Where can I get the new information (read: knowledge and skills) I need?*

Find someone to bounce ideas off of. Form a mastermind group. Everyone knows someone who has a talent or skill that can complement their own. Put your minds together to create what you want. Instead of assuming that we are in this alone and that no one can help us, we should continually ask ourselves, *"Who can help me and how can I help them?"*

When change comes (and it's coming), it's up to each of us to relate decisively to that change, rather than passively allowing the change to take us where it may. We have the choice of taking control of our actions and the situations, and creating progress.

We'll never know the outcomes unless we try. We can always revamp and act again. Better to fail from making an effort than from inertia. *Why not try?*

Do the next right thing, or at least do something that you believe is the next right thing. Better to do the right thing wrong, than the wrong thing right. The key is to DO something. Learn something. Try something.

Act. Get rolling.

Stop, BOP, and Roll your way to working and winning.

Be Progress.

Ponder & Progress: Finding Progress in Change

1. What changes in the past have you transitioned into personal progress?

2. What changes are reshaping your industry?

3. What changes are happening in your personal life?

4. How will you find the progress in the change?

5. What do you need to stop doing or thinking to start progressing?

6. What feelings are you letting get in your way?

7. How can you become more open to progress?

8. What do you need to "unlearn" to progress?

9. Where can you get reliable information?

10. When will you make action the way you roll?

> "Weep not that the world changes – did it keep a stable, changeless state, 'twere cause indeed to weep."
> -- *William Cullen Bryant*

The Progress Challenge

Committing to Progress

We Don't Have to Do Anything, But We Can't Do Nothing.

Ever call up a buddy and ask, *"What are you doing?"* and they said, *"Nothing."* You can't do "nothing." Doing nothing requires taking heavy medication. Actually, taking heavy medication is still doing something. Sleeping is doing something. So is staring into space; so is flossing your teeth; so is scratching your arm; so is eating a plate of lima beans; so is waiting in the dentist's waiting room. We are always investing our time somewhere for some reason. We might not connect with the reasons consciously, but we are always doing something.

> **"Doing nothing is not as easy as it looks. You have to be careful, because the idea of doing anything could easily lead to doing something, which would cut into your nothing and force you to have to drop everything."**
> -- Jerry Seinfeld

We have each said to ourselves at some point, *"Why am I doing this?"* Consciously or unconsciously, we choose to do what we believe to be the best option at the time. We may even know consciously that the activity is not *good* for us but still we do it. There are reasons. They are our reasons. We may not be able to vocalize them, or even wrap our minds around them, but we have reasons for the actions we take. The action may not be what we <u>wished</u> we would have <u>wanted</u> to take. Still, we chose to act (based on the circumstances and anticipated consequences). That is what personal regret is: wishing we'd have wanted to do something differently.

Committing to Progress

When we look back upon actions we have regretted, we find that, at the time, we thought that taking the action would help us attain some mixture of pleasure, peace of mind, profit, prestige, pain avoidance, and power. We regret the action because we did not receive the Ps that we expected, and/or because our actions deprived someone else of those good outcomes.

Have you ever heard someone say, "I don't have a choice"? Not true. We always have a choice, usually several. The choices may not be enjoyable, safe, or even legal, but there are always choices. Every choice has consequences. Maybe we view the consequences as unpalatably negative for us, but we do have choices. The choices might not be choice choices, but there are always choices from which to choose *(that was a fun sentence to write).*

We don't have many **have to's**.
We don't *have to* kiss our spouse.
We don't *have to* exercise; we don't *have to* pray.
We don't *have to* smile, or even brush our teeth.
We don't *have to* sleep or pay our mortgage.
We don't *have to* feed our pets or hug our kids.
We don't *have to* pay for our kids' higher education (or for our pet's higher education, for that matter).
We don't *have to* eat.
You say, "Wait a minute, Deano. We **have to** eat."
Are there people who chose not to eat? Yes.
What has happened to them? They died (painfully). It's still a choice. (If you know me, you know I choose to eat, and hug my kids, and to pray, for that matter.)

We do not *have to* pay our income tax. The consequences may include us going to jail but that is our choice.

We do not *have to* stop at stop lights. The consequences may include injuring ourselves and others – again, our choice. We do not *have to* work. We've sold ourselves *(most would say rightfully)* on the idea that the benefits of working outweigh the benefits of not working.
I asked a group I was working with once:
"Do you have to work?"
Somebody yelled out, *"You do if you don't want to live in a tent."*
I said, *"Are there people who choose to live in tents?"*
They responded, *"Yeah. But I don't want to live in a tent."*
I said, *"Exactly."*

These are choices that we are making. There is power in that. **At each moment, we make decisions based on what we believe will help us feel the *Six Ps of Progress* – in the short term or long term.** As an example, let's take an activity that most people would say they wish they didn't **have to** do – mowing the lawn.
Why mow the lawn?
- Maybe we want to have a good-looking yard like the neighbors do, and don't want to look like dirtbags. (*Prestige; Pain avoidance*)
- Maybe it gives us a sense of accomplishment and a chance to think. (*Peace of Mind, Pleasure*)
- Maybe we believe lawn mowing offers exercise. (*Pleasure, Pain Avoidance*)
- Maybe we don't want to get fined by the city. (*Pain avoidance*)
- Maybe a significant other "told" us to. (*Pain avoidance of not doing what significant other wants; Pleasure from pleasing significant other*)
- Maybe we would rather keep our money than pay someone else to mow it. (*Profit, Pain Avoidance*)

Committing to Progress

How we judge the results is subjective. Having a well-groomed lawn offers progress for some. For others, amassing a noteworthy collection of vintage lipstick holders offers progress. There is always a result, an outcome. *We cannot not accomplish something.* Some shift in feeling attends everything that we do. There is a new normal. It may be only ever so slightly new, but it's new.

> There is *some* profit in having a garage sale.
> There is *some* power in punching someone.
> There is *some* pleasure in eating a bag of *Pringles*.

(I know it is not a *bag* of Pringles but what is it -- a cardboard sphere of Pringles? What? A *tube* of Pringles, I guess.)

We may not like or care for what is achieved, but there are outcomes and consequences – and these outcomes affect our next action.

Did the action (eating that sandwich, working for that company, using that wireless company, reading that book, wearing those shoes, buying that house) result in us feeling enough pleasure, peace of mind, profit, prestige, and power?

Did the action help us avoid enough pain?

There are outcomes for both parties when someone chooses to utilize our products and services. There are outcomes when someone decides not to utilize our products and services. This is also extremely subjective. We value achievements, as well as gauge success, based on whether the time and effort invested in the activity help us feel *enough* of the Six Ps of Progress.

We can't choose nothing. Choose Progress.

Defining Your Parameters for Progress

*What does **Working and Winning** mean to you?*
What would bring you the most pleasure, peace of mind, profit, prestige, power, and pain avoidance?
What are your goals? Why?
What do you want out of life?

These important questions are far too often overlooked. I don't presume to know what you should want out of your day or your life, but I do know that our actions are futile if we don't know what *we really want*.

The following Parameters of Progress exercise can be unnerving because we don't ordinarily take the time to think like this. There is so much going on in our immediate day-to-day lives that we don't give ourselves a chance to reflect on our lives relative to the big picture.

The Four-Minute, Four-Step Personal Parameters for Progress Exercise

Step One
Take a piece of paper and write today's date at the top but add 15 years. Then write, *"Today I am ..."* and write your age but again add 15 years. (Scary, I know.)

Step Two
Think of all you want to have accomplished within the next 15 years. Take a breath and write nonstop for four solid minutes. Write down everything you want to have done with your life in those 15 years.

Committing to Progress

Imagine that whatever you get down on the paper will happen, and what you do not get on the paper won't. List experiences you want to have enjoyed, people you want to have helped, things you have acquired, qualities of character you have internalized. Include the things you want to stop happening, bad habits or bad feelings. You are the artist. Paint the picture. Dare to dream.

Questions to Ponder for Defining Your Parameters for Progress

How do you envision your next 15 years?
What do you want to have accomplished?
What do you want to have seen?
Want to get married, or get married again? Have children?
Spend more time with your children?
Put your kids through college? Open a pet store?
What cities and countries do you want to have visited?
Maybe you want to visit the New 7 Wonders of the World?
Want to stop drinking, smoking, eating fried foods?
What musicians do you want to have seen in concert?
Maybe you want to be in a play or ride in a helicopter?
Climb a mountain, run a marathon, bench 200 pounds?
Earn your master's degree?
Earn a black belt in Tang Soo Do?
Want to write a book or learn guitar?
Learn to scuba dive, box, or fly a plane?
Any people you want to have helped? Who?
Want to donate to charities? Which charities?
Care for your parents in their old age?
What do you want?

**Life offers Endless Choices.
Which are Progress and which are Change to YOU?
What are your Parameters of Progress?**

Committing to Progress

Step Three
Estimate how much time it would take to achieve each item on your list if you started today.
A month? Six months? One year? Five years? Fifteen years? Hint: Fifteen years is the max.

Step Four
Go back to the top of the page and circle the year (plus 15) and your age (plus 15). Those are the only two facts on the page. Fifteen years from now you will be that age.

The rest is up to you.

Be Progress.

Something Wonderful to know
The NEW 7 Wonders of the World, which were officially announced at a ceremony in Lisbon, Portugal, on July 7, 2007 (07.07.07), are:
Chichén Itzá, Mexico
Christ the Redeemer, Brazil
Machu Picchu, Peru
Great Wall of China
Petra, Jordan
The Roman Coliseum, Italy
The Taj Mahal, India

The Great Pyramid of Giza in Egypt is the only one of the original "Seven Wonders of the Ancient World" that still exists. It was decided that the Great Pyramid would not be included as one of the new Seven Wonders to offer it special recognition as the only remaining original World Wonder.

An Introduction to Progress-Based Goal-Crafting

To work and win in this world of change we must dedicate ourselves to _crafting_ personal and organizational goals that are so attractive, so alluring, that we are compelled to continually make choices that move us toward their accomplishment.

As a noun, <u>craft</u> can mean an object or machine designed for a journey, like a ship or an airplane.

As a verb, <u>craft</u> can mean to make or manufacture with skill and careful attention to detail.

A <u>goal</u> is the aim, the objective, the purpose, the point.

Goal-crafting is the practice of creating personal and organizational targets that are so clear, so detailed, so sound, so enticing and leakproof that they actually become tools or vessels in our journey to their accomplishment.

Our lives and organizations will surely change without well-crafted goals, but it is doubtful that they will progress.

Well-crafted, progress-based goals do not merely remind us of the desired destination; they help create the conditions and environment needed for their achievement. They propel us into forward-focused action and strengthen our resolve to work and win in a world of change.

A Progress Agent's Six Rules for Goal-Crafting

1. Progress-Crafted Goals Are Written and Visualized.
Written goals crystallize thinking, enhance commitment, and help identify the strong reasons that propel the strong actions. Having goals in writing gives them weight and more importance: for whatever reason, not only the conscious but the subconscious mind takes them much more seriously. Written goals are also vital when developing a course of action.

> "If a man knows not what harbor he seeks, any wind is the right wind."
> -- *Lucius Annaeus Seneca*

The mind will not reach for achievement until it has clear objectives. Writing and frequently rereading goals turns on the "Can Do" switch in our brain, and the power to accomplish the goal begins to flow. Goals that are written, read, rewritten, rephrased, and reread get impressed into our subconscious mind. We may not know exactly how to go about achieving our goals, and our conscious mind may not even think them possible, but if we write out our goals and visualize their accomplishment every day, our subconscious mind will work to make them a reality.

Myth alert: The "Yale Study of Goals" is often cited as a testament to the power of written goals. However, most scholars doubt the 1953 "study" ever took place. The so-called study claimed to have found that the 3% of Yale graduates who had written goals at the time of graduation were worth more financially twenty years later than the remaining 97% combined. Too bad the "YSG" is probably an urban legend, because properly written goals are actually

Committing to Progress – Goal-Crafting

vital, and today it is estimated that fewer than 5% of us have properly written goals. Let's get that percentage up by "getting down with" writing our goals down.

2. Progress-Crafted Goals Connect to Personal Progress. Plainly put, each person involved in a goal's achievement must believe there is something favorable in it for him or her. We are unlikely to work toward a goal that we can not personalize as positive for us. For a goal to actually become a tool in its own achievement, it must generate genuine excitement when we envision its accomplishment. *Why and how does the goal mean Progress for those who must act?*

Often, individuals must make an organizational goal their own, as in a new technology rollout, reorganization, or a merger. To get all team members (including ourselves) psyched and committed to the organization's goal, we need to dig into how the goal's achievement will benefit all involved (via job security, bonuses, flex time, exciting new projects, raises, promotions, shorter commute, less stress, etc.).

If team members believe that the potential for progress is worth the effort, they will more readily take on challenges in support of the organization's goals. When highlighting the reasons behind the goal, include the Six Ps of Progress.

Whether the goal is meeting sales quota, buying a new boat, becoming more efficient in customer-service calls, or finishing a financial report, we must find ways to make the goal progress for us in some way. With that personal lodestar ever in sight, we stay committed to reaching the goal. *Why we want to achieve a goal is far more important than the goal itself.*

Committing to Progress – Goal-Crafting

3. Progress-Crafted Goals Are Stated in Present Tense.
Stating goals in the present tense tells our subconscious mind that we are committed – that the goals will not remain forever stuck in a future tense – as in, *I WILL be wealthy.* Our mind takes ownership, sees the goal as an actuality (rather than a potentiality) – *I AM wealthy* – and works toward its realization.

> "Victorious warriors win first and then go to war, while defeated warriors go to war first and then seek to win."
> -- *Sun Tzu*

The subconscious mind chooses a path of least resistance. If we write, *"I will be debt-free,"* the subconscious mind does not act, because the "will" postpones the goal's achievement to some indefinite time in the future. When we craft a goal as if it were already achieved, already true, our minds want to make it happen. Examples:

Daily, I am ...	*I weigh___ with a ___waist.*
I know how to...	*My family and I are...*
I own...	*I feel...*

Well-crafted goals, stated in the present tense, serve as affirmations. Think of affirmations as personalized powerful ads that you tell yourself over and over again about yourself and your life. Get over any weird thoughts you might have about affirmations – we all use them. We have lived our whole lives making affirmations. Unfortunately, affirmations are often self-critical and self-limiting:

I am fat.	*I am a lousy speller.*
I am not a good salesman.	*I am always tired.*
I know nothing about investments.	*I'm destined to be poor.*

Be careful about everything you say to yourself, or think to yourself, about yourself, because you'll end up being right. As Luigi Pirandello noted some time ago, "Così è (se vi pare)" – Right you are (if you think you are).

> **Your brain is a terrible thing
> to use against yourself.**

4. Progress-Crafted Goals Are Detailed and Measured.
We are able to measure and track progress only toward goals that are detailed and specific. It is imperative that we craft goals with precise and vivid outcomes so that we can be sure we are progressing and not merely changing.

A vague, general, or conflicted goal produces vague actions and vague results. A specific goal produces specific actions and specific results. The more information we can give our subconscious mind about our intentions – *our wants, our goals* – the clearer the right next steps become, and the more focused our actions will be. It is fine if the goal takes many words to map out. The key is to crystallize our intentions.

For example, *"I have a new job"* is generic, not very helpful, and certainly not very inspiring. Most of us could get a *new job* within a week, if not a day. It probably would not be a job that matched our skills, paid well, or that we even liked, but we could get *a job*. So be darn sure to specify:

In what industry?   *What position and responsibilities?*
What pay range?   *What benefits, 401K, vacation?*
How much travel?   *How long commute?*
Company car?   *Work from home?*
What kind of boss (if any), and coworkers?

Committing to Progress – Goal-Crafting

Our "specs" can go on and on. Generic goals do little to propel us to action. Yes, it takes time, but it is vital that we craft our goals in as much detail as possible. It is perfectly fine to rewrite the goal, refine it, add to it, mess with it.

Becoming almost ridiculously particular about what we want, and *why* we want it, helps create the inspiration that propels us to progress toward our goals – instead of focusing attention on the countless other options of how we could invest our time and energy.

5. Progress-Crafted Goals Are Positively Worded.
Words hold great power. They have since "the beginning." Crafted goals should focus our conscious and subconscious minds on future progress, not past problems and limitations. Therefore, we should craft goals that focus on what we want, not on what we don't.

Any words or phrases that have negative connotations perpetuate frustration, worry, and regret because they remind us of past weaknesses or failures. In turn, this can create a mental block that limits our pattern of thought and behavior. It is helpful to become aware of when we're using defeatist words like *can not, do not, will not, never.* We need to rephrase our goal statements, eliminating any negative words and using believable, positive words.

Instead of writing, *"I don't eat junk food,"* write, *"I am a healthy eater. I eat foods that are good for me."* Then list healthy foods and why healthy choices are good for you.

Instead of writing, *"I will not stay up late, oversleep, and be late to work,"* write, *"I go to bed by 10:30 p.m. each night and am on time for work each day."* Then list five ways in which early to bed, early to rise, makes you healthy, wealthy, and wise. There are three ways right there. *Thanks, Ben Franklin!*

Crafting goals from a positive perspective raises our expectations and encourages empowering thought processes. We get our subconscious to work for us, opening up our options and making things seem possible and more doable.

The subconscious mind does not judge or argue; it only carries out instructions. The more positive the imagery we sow in our conscious and subconscious minds, the more positive results we will reap.

6. Progress-Crafted Goals Have an Achievement Date. Achievement dates are vital for measuring and tracking our progress. Many of us waste a great deal of time talking about what we want to do, or to have, or to become, someday. *Someday is not a day of the week.* *

Without an end date there is no strong reason to take strong action today. Having a specific time frame gives us the push, the prod, the sense of urgency to get moving. *Achievement date or procrastinate?* Set one and get moving before it's too late. (Hey, that rhymes.)

Without a date for accomplishment, we have only crafted a wishy-washy wish which floats around. We never get moving because we feel we can start at any time. A realistic time frame helps reel the goal in and make it real. Grounding our goals within a realistic time frame gets the fire burning and sets our subconscious mind in motion.

Committing to Progress – Goal-Crafting

Many of us have so many goals that we end up pursuing two dozen of them poorly, rather than three or four with laser-like focus and unflagging effort. Establishing achievement dates for our goals helps us decide which ones warrant the majority of today's time and energy.

Often it turns out that we have underestimated the true time, effort, and knowledge required to accomplish our goals. We run out of patience and passion, or lose sight of the goal's purpose. Most of our goals can be met if they have realistic achievement dates and we work to stay committed to them. If we don't achieve our goal within our time frame, we can always set a new achievement date.

> **"The greatest danger for most of us is not that our aim is too high and we miss it, but that it is too low and we reach it."**
> -- *Michelangelo*

Craft and commit to progress-based goals.

Be Progress.

* *Someday Is Not a Day of the Week* is the title of an insightful, motivating, and eye-opening children's book by Denise Brennan-Nelson. I recommend it highly.

Committing to Progress

The hardest aspect of goal achievement is not in crafting a goal or even in knowing how to achieve it. The real challenge is staying connected to the passion and understanding of WHY. Understanding the reasons behind our goal channels the passion in the right direction, or at least in *some* direction.

We initiate actions because, *in that moment*, we believe those actions will bring us the *Six Ps of Progress* with more intensity than any other option – short-term or long-term. Whatever goal we craft, it needs to *LOOM LARGE* in our mind for us to continually work toward achieving it.

Will reaching your crafted goal bring you more pleasure, peace of mind, profit, prestige, pain avoidance and power than any other actions you could take? Why or why not?

This concept is simple, but not easy. It is hard and even impossible to practice 24/7. It is very common to start our day committed to doing *this* and to not doing *that,* only to end up that day doing *that* and not doing *this*. It's not that we forgot, or got confused. As the day wore on, what we were initially committed to shifted, and other things became more attractive, took precedence, seemed somehow more pressing to us.

We might stop taking steps toward a particular goal, but we are always moving toward outcomes that we believe will help us feel peace of mind, pleasure, profit, prestige, pain avoidance, and power.

Committing to Progress

Though constantly reminded of *good* ways we could and should invest our time and money, it is easy to get led away from our goals. Our heads can be turned by the immediate gratification we would receive by taking some other action, or even agreeing to pursue someone else's goals. There are some benefits, be they ever so humble, to pretty much every activity.

Are there benefits in eating a jelly donut?
 Pleasure (by the ton) and short-term pain avoidance.
Are there benefits in not eating a jelly donut?
 Pleasure, pain avoidance, power, prestige, and profit.

Are there benefits in spending twelve hours a day at your job or running your business?
Are there benefits in taking a day or a week off?

Are there benefits in getting up early in the morning?
Are there benefits in sleeping in?

Are there benefits to you in handling everything yourself?
Are there benefits in delegating?

Are there benefits in working out?
Are there benefits in not working out?

Commitment is a moment-by-moment decision. Reminding ourselves about the pleasure, peace of mind, profit, and prestige we will enjoy, and the pain we will avoid by accomplishing our crafted goals, generates the commitment and motivation to do, reach, and act.

"With the power of conviction, there is no sacrifice."
-- *Pat Benatar*

Committing to Progress

We live in a drive-thru society. <u>Beware the lure of Insta-Progress.</u> The opportunity for some level of instant gratification is all around us. If we feel the need for a little bit of pleasure, *boom!* There's a fast-food restaurant right around the corner. *Want to avoid some pain?* Just flip on the tube.

We are offered countless ways to take the easy road to some lesser form of progress. Without personal, healthy, short- and long-range personalized goals, we are at the mercy of any person or circumstance with a little weight, anything with some decent-sounding *whys*. **The Six Ps of Progress attached to our goals must shine more brightly in our minds than the benefits of anything else we could do at that moment.**

Don't remind yourself about a goal.
Remind yourself of the benefits of the goal.

Don't tell or remind prospects about your product.
Share with them how your products help them to progress.

Don't remind sales professionals of their sales goals.
Remind them about the money they will make, or the trips they will earn by reaching their sales goals.

Don't remind team members about the change needed.
Remind them of the progress achieved by making the change.

It helps to advertise the benefits of your goals. Post these benefits someplace where you will see them. Effective advertising campaigns don't show us a product, they show how the product or service will positively affect our life – i.e., help us avoid pain, or gain pleasure.

Committing to Progress

Ads don't just pop up at one time. Advertisers <u>continually</u> remind us about the benefits of their products and services. Ad agencies know the power of repetition, repetition, repetition. We must continually remind all involved why the goal *(company goal, sales goal, safety goal, or purely personal goal)* is important to progress.

How can you advertise your crafted goals?

Maybe you could "Carrey" the reasons around. When actor Jim Carrey was just starting out in show business, he wrote himself a ten-million-dollar check for acting services rendered. He carried this check in his wallet for years as he auditioned around Hollywood – to remind himself WHY.

**We don't forget about our goals;
we forget WHY they are our goals.**

**Our goals must be the tastiest goodies
on the smorgasbord of life.**

Be Progress.

Ponder & Progress: Committing to Progress

1. Will your crafted goal's achievement bring you pleasure? More pleasure than anything else you could choose to do with your time?

2. Will your crafted goal's achievement bring you peace of mind? More peace than anything else you could choose to do?

3. Will your crafted goal's achievement bring you profit? More profit than anything else you could choose to do?

4. Will your crafted goal's achievement bring you prestige? More prestige than anything else you could choose to do?

5. Will your crafted goal's achievement help you avoid pain? What pain will you be likely to feel if you do not accomplish that goal? What is more painful -- the discipline now, or the regret later?

6. Will your crafted goal's achievement bring you power? More power than anything else you could choose to do?

7. What habits will you have to break to achieve this goal? Why will you break them?

8. What habits will you have to establish?

Two Most Important Questions:
9. Are you committed to this goal? Why?

10. How are you continually reminding yourself of the reasons behind your crafted goal?

Progress Takes Persistence

> "Nothing in the world can take the place of persistence."
> -- *Calvin Coolidge*

Personal, professional, and social progress demands persistent action. The greatest goals, ideas, plans, and skills in the world are useless unless they are combined with a generous amount of persistence. Persistence is a byproduct of passion. Passion leads to a zest in the pursuit. To keep the passion, we must constantly remind ourselves of the benefits we are expecting from our efforts.

News flash
Goals <u>can</u> be achieved *without a plan.* It will most likely take us much longer, but we will eventually progress if we stay *committed.* The dangerous thing about not having a plan is that the longer it takes to progress toward a goal, the more likely we are to search out or give in to other ways to try to feel the *Six Ps of Progress.* Note that I said *other* ways, not better ways. And I said *try to feel,* not feel.

Without a plan, we are likely to get discouraged and give up. "Losing sight of the goal" means that it has not been defined clearly enough, and/or not held on to long enough, to be realized. A plan helps us achieve our crafted goals faster and more efficiently, without wasting resources or pulling our hair out.

Committing to Progress - Persistence

Let's say I wanted to travel:
> **From:** Columbus, Ohio *(girlhood home of Erma Louise Fiste, later known as Erma Bombeck).*
> **To:** Hannibal, Missouri *(boyhood town of Samuel Clemens, later known as Mark Twain).*

Maybe I'm hoping to start a tour business, highlighting the childhood towns of America's wittiest. Anyway, I'm ready to roll, and my wallet's bulging with fifties, so I get into the car and buckle up. I have everything I need, except for a plan: no map, no GPS, no particular itinerary. I have a full tank of gas, so I turn the key and drive. I am committed to getting to Hannibal.

Will I eventually get to Hannibal?

Yes, if I am persistent, I will *eventually* make my way to Hannibal. It might take me a week, and I may run out of money, have to sell the car and then hitchhike the last 75 miles, but if I'm persistent, I will eventually get to Hannibal.

A plan would certainly help me get there a lot faster, without having to ask a bunch of people for directions, without running out of money, or hitchhiking. However, it is not the plan that makes achievement possible. It is persistent action. And action is initiated and sustained by strong, internalized reasons.

> ***Don't get me wrong.***
> ***I am a firm believer in planning.***
> ***But the best-laid plans of mice and men***
> ***will not take us where we are not***
> ***committed to going.***

Committing to Progress - Persistence

Keeping our thoughts constantly on the reasons behind our goals is the stimulus that keeps us committed and able to dispense with setbacks quickly, and to decisively redirect our efforts.

"*Nana korobi ya oki*" is a popular Japanese saying that vividly expresses the importance of persistence, despite setbacks. As the proverb teaches, the eventual winners are those who "fall down seven times, get up eight."

> **"Making miracles is hard work.
> Most people give up before they happen."**
> *-- Sheryl Crow*

Every moment that we focus on the strong reasons that have inspired our goals, the closer we are to taking determined action toward their achievement. The key is to not let reasons for pursuing other goals steal our attention, or become more compelling. We must keep our focus *(and our employees', customers', and prospects' focus)* on the Six Ps of Progress that will be felt in accomplishing the goal.

The Progress Challenge Riddle *(a classic)*
If there are five frogs on a log and three decide to jump off, how many frogs are still on the log?
Answer: *Five. Deciding is not doing.*

Decided to make sales calls?
We may have decided to make a sales call, and it may even play out very nicely in our minds, but until we pick up the phone and dial, we are not making sales calls.

And we can't let a misguided desire for perfection stop us. We don't have to be perfect to *Be Progress*. We can always improve our technique, improve our plan and our actions.

Progress does not demand perfection, only persistence.

Things can and do go wrong. Missed opportunities should not be allowed to become big emotional "downers." Self-pity is not part of a Progress Agent's makeup. We must reframe setbacks to our advantage. Most "successful" people say they learned more from their failures than their successes because they were eager to learn what went wrong and to avoid repeating it.

Being persistent does not mean being bullheaded. If what we're trying isn't working, we must take a fresh approach. Consider that by eliminating another idea that didn't work, the path to progress became clearer. When things go wrong, we can let Thomas Edison light our way. Asked if he was discouraged after thousands of attempts at creating a viable light bulb had failed, he replied: *"Why would I feel like a failure? And why would I ever give up? I now know definitively over 9,000 ways that an electric light bulb will not work."* Make time on a regular basis to revise the plan. Creating a feedback loop is vital – even if we're the only ones in the loop.

Fill days with action toward crafted goals. Start and, if we get sidetracked, we must acknowledge that the reasons for pursuing some other goal or goals have become stronger in our mind. Then is the time to ask: *Why?*

Committing to Progress - Persistence

If the promise of our goals no longer propels us to action, we need to do a gut check.

Are they still our goals?

Are the reasons strong enough to propel us to persistent action?

> **"What man actually needs is not a tensionless state but rather the striving and struggling for some goal worthy of him. What he needs is not the discharge of tension at any cost, but the call of a potential meaning waiting to be fulfilled by him."**
> *-- Viktor Frankl*

Each step toward a goal is progress. It is powerful for us to appreciate all that we're doing to stay on track, and to express our gratitude to those who are helping and supporting us. Find ways to enjoy the journey. Pat yourself on the back. Reward yourself. *These are <u>our lives</u> we are talking about here.*

Go. Do. Progress takes persistence.

Be Progress.

Committing to Progress - Persistence

Progress Challenge Quote Quiz
Who said it? Bombeck or Twain?

1. "God created man, but I could do better."

2. "There are people who put their dreams in a little box and say, 'Yes, I've got dreams, of course I've got dreams.' Then they put the box away and bring it out once in a while to look in it, and yep, they're still there."

3. "There is a thin line that separates laughter and pain, comedy and tragedy, humor and hurt."

[*For the answers, turn to page 202*]

Committing to Progress - Persistence

Ponder & Progress: Progress Takes Persistence

1. How are you reminding yourself of the benefits of your goals?

2. What steps have you taken today toward your goal?

3. What actions could you take today that would be progress toward your crafted goals?

4. What activities will you trim back or cut out to achieve your goals?

5. What do you need to do, learn, or become to progress?

6. How will you begin acquiring the new skills you need to progress?

7. Which new people do you need to build relationships with?

8. What is working? What have you learned?

9. What new obstacles are there?

10. How will you become more persistent?

> "I'm tired of dreaming. I'm into doing at the moment. It's, like, let's only have goals that we can go after."
> -- *Bono*

Answers to the
Progress Challenge Quote Quiz
from page 200.

Who said it -- Bombeck or Twain?

All three of the quotes are from Erma Bombeck.
To balance the scale, here are three from Mark Twain that could easily have been Erma's.

"Human pride is not worthwhile; there is always something lying in wait to take the wind out of it." -- MT

"The dictionary is the only place where success comes before work." -- MT

"Thousands of geniuses live and die undiscovered -- either by themselves or by others." -- MT

The Little Mind That Could

I was listening to my elder daughter, Sofia, reading Wally Piper's classic *The Little Engine That Could* to her younger sister, Ella, one night and it occurred to me what a powerful little story it is. In his book, Mr. Piper shares the story of a little red engine pulling a train "filled full of good things for boys and girls" on the other side of a mountain.

When the little red engine breaks down, a toy clown hops off the little train and starts asking larger passing trains if they will help.

The first two trains refuse to help because they feel they are too big and important to pull toys and goodies.

A rusty third train relates that he is too old and tired to help, and chugs away saying, *"I can not. I can not. I can not."*

Finally, a little blue engine passes by and stops immediately when she sees the clown waving. The little engine's first words are, *"What is the matter, my friends?"*

The clown relays the challenge, and the little blue engine explains that she has never been over the mountain. She then sees the tears in the dolls' eyes and thinks of the good little girls and boys who will not have any toys to play with or good food to eat unless she helps. She looks at the mountain and says, *"I think I can. I think I can. I think I can."*

The Progress Challenge

The little blue engine hitches herself to the little train and starts tugging and pulling and pulling and tugging. Slowly, the train moves forward.

> **"Puff, puff, chug, chug, went the Little Blue Engine.**
> **'I think I can. I think I can. I think I can.**
> **I think I can. I think I can. I think I can.**
> **I think I can. I think I can. I think I can.'"**
> -- *from* The Little Engine That Could
> *by Wally Piper*

Up they go, ever so slowly to the top of the mountain. When they reach the top, the toys cheer. After coming down the mountain and unhitching the train, the little blue engine chugs away, saying happily, *"I thought I could. I thought I could. I thought I could."*

The conviction that we have the power to progress is a major key to progressing. Remember, *our brains want to be right.* Whatever the mind believes, it will work to make true. But, the little blue engine didn't say, *"I think I can,"* only one time. She said it over and over and over and over. Repetition, repetition, repetition.

What do you think that little blue engine will say next time she is asked to pull a train over a mountain?
Will she say, "I think I can"?
I think not. She will say, *"Yes, I can."*

Also, the little blue engine did not say, *"I think I can,"* and then glide away. She said it and immediately hitched herself to the little train and started tugging and pulling and pulling and tugging. To progress in this world of change, there must be ACTION. No dallying!

The Progress Challenge

The little blue engine had to tug and pull to reach her goal. *Will some of the progressive action steps that you and your company need to take to climb that mountain and reach your crafted goals be painful?* **Yes.** Again, consider: *What is more painful to you, discipline or regret?*

Finally, the little blue engine had strong reasons. She saw the tears in the dolls' eyes and considered the little children, who would not have any toys or good food to eat unless she helped. She would feel pain if she didn't help, and would gain pleasure, prestige, and power if she did.

Develop strong reasons for taking strong action. Remind yourself often of the personal benefits that reaching your and your company's goals will have for your life. Help others develop strong reasons, so they too choose to take strong actions.

Define your Parameters for Progress.
Commit to well-crafted, progress-based goals.
Stop Changing and Start Progressing.
Uncover others' Parameters for Progress.
Earn and Maintain Customer Loyalty.
Be a BAM and Believe you can help others progress.
Stop, BOP, and Roll.
Focus on Being Progress – not being perfect.
Believe in yourself. Chug. Chug. Puff. Puff.

Progress is a step forward. Take today's step. To change is human; to progress, divine.

Meet the Progress Challenge.

Be Progress.

Index

abstinence, as Holy Virtue, 117
achievement dates, 186–187.
    See also time management
actions
    consequences affecting, 174
    defined, 30
    reasons for, 31–32
    taking the first step and, 204–205
advertising, of goals, 191–192
affirmations, 136, 183
alcohol, and bottom line, 141
Ali, Muhammad, 159
American Institute for Stress, 129
American Medical Association, 129
Anderson, Greg, 132
appearance, and organization, 78
Aristotle, 115
attitude. *See* perspective, positive
Aurelius, Marcus, 130
awards, 85, 89–91, 148.
    See also prestige

balance
    choices in achieving, 125–127
    competition and, 122–123
    excess preventing, 123–124
    internalizing for, 124–125
    motives in finding, 121–122
    self-assessment, 128
BAMs. *See* Business Attraction Magnets
Barnes, Dorothy, 48–49
Barnes, Robert, 48–49
Barrett, Colleen, 65
Battista, O.A., 86
Bavarian Grill, 86
Be Open to Progress (BOP), 161–163.
    See also Stop, BOP, and Roll

Beecher, Henry Ward, 138
Benatar, Pat, 190
Berger, Thomas, 75
Bethlehem Steel Company, 145
Big PHAT Goals program, 97–101
blame, assigning, 157–158
Blanchard, Ken, 52
Blockbuster, 15
Bombeck, Erma, 196, 200, 202
bombs, dropping, 162–163
Bono, 201
Boone, Louis E., 144
BOP (Be Open to Progress), 161–163.
    See also Stop, BOP, and Roll
breathing, deep, 138
Brennan-Nelson, Denise, *Someday Is Not a Day of the Week,* 187
Brillat-Savarin, Anthelme, 141
Brooks, Mel, 138
Bryant, William Cullen, 168
budgeting, as stress defense, 140
Buffett, Jimmy, 53
Buscaglia, Leo, 52
Business Attraction Magnets (BAMs).
    See also profit
    buzz-worthiness of, 74
    changing environment and, 73–74
    empathy of, 80–81
    listening by, 77–78
    open-ended questions from, 75–76
    price versus cost and, 82
    relationships of, 80
    respecting time and structure, 78–79
buzz-worthiness, 74

Calgon, 94
card games, and customer care payoff, 57
Carnegie, Dale, *How to Win Friends and Influence People,* 36–37

Carrey, Jim, 192
challenge, defined, 7
change
    finding progress in, 168
        (*see also* Stop, BOP, and Roll)
    progress versus, 23, 24–26, 27, 52
change management, Progress Leadership versus, 35–38
chastity, as Holy Virtue, 117
choice
    in achieving balance, 125–127
    power of, 103
    Six Ps of Progress, 172–174, 189–191
    in stress management, 132
Clemens, Samuel, 196, 200, 202
commitment. *See also* goal-crafting
    Parameters of Progress in, 175–177
    procrastination versus, 158
    reinforcing, 189–192
company side of change management, 37
comparisons, 122–123. *See also* balance
competition, 122–123. *See also* balance
compliments, 86. *See also* prestige
concentration camps, 108–109
Confucius, 166
consequences, in delegating, 148
conviction, power of, 204
Coolidge, Calvin, 195
cost
    price versus, 82
    of stress, 130 (*see also* stress)
Covey, Stephen, 30, 124
*Cracking the Networking CODE:
4 Steps, Priceless Business Relationships*
(Lindsay), 80.
craft, defined, 177. *See also* goal-crafting
Croce, Jim, 121
Crow, Sheryl, 95, 197
culture, organizational,
    pleasure from, 11–12, 64–65
customer advocates, 59
customer care. *See also* peace of mind
    beneficiaries of good, 55–56
    defining way of, 60
    describing levels of, 57–58
    customer disservice as, 57

    losing sight of, 57
    perspective on recipients of, 58–59, 60
    pleasure from, 17 (*see also* Donut Man)
customer disservice, 57, 64
customer service. *See* customer care
customer-service reps, 59
customers
    defining, 59, 60
    dissatisfied, 57, 64
    Southwest Airlines view of, 11–12

debt, as stressor, 140
delegating, 148–149
Deming, W. Edwards, 52, 60
detail, in goal-crafting, 184–185
diet, stress management and, 141
diligence, as Holy Virtue, 117
displeasure, customers feeling, 57, 64
Do it now habit, 166
Donut Man, 15–17, 67–68
drill sergeant, 97–101
dropping bombs, 162–163
Drucker, Peter, 152
Dyer, Wayne, 52

Edison, Thomas, 198
education, as source of power, 104
effectiveness, versus efficiency, 149–150
efficiency, versus effectiveness, 149–150
80-20 Rule, 150
Einstein, Albert, 128, 142, 161
Eisenberg, Larry, 54
email, checking, 151
Emerson, Ralph Waldo, 158
empathy, practicing, 80–81
employees
    in change management, 37
    corporate culture affecting, 11, 12, 64, 65
    partnering with organizations, 41–43, 44
    Southwest Airlines view of, 11–12
enemies from within, 31
envy, as Deadly Sin, 117
excess, balance affected by, 123–124
exercise, as stress defense, 139

Facebook, 26

failure
    fear of, 158, 166
    learning from, 198
Fast Company, 29
feedback loops, 198
feelings, versus wants, 159
Ferriss, Timothy,
    The 4-Hour Workweek, 150
fight-or-flight mode, 131
Fillmore, Millard, 23
Fiste, Erma Louise, 196, 200, 202
flexibility, 142, 162
The 4-Hour Workweek (Ferriss), 150
Four-Minute, Four-Step Personal Parameters for Progress Exercise, 175–177
Frankl, Viktor. *See also* logotherapy
    about, 38, 48, 107, 112
    Man's Search for Meaning, 108–109
    paradoxical intent technique, 141
    on persistence, 199
    on power, 103, 104, 105
    Say Yes to Life in Spite of Everything: A Psychologist Experiences the Concentration Camp, 108–109
    Frankl Institute of Logotherapy, 48
Franklin, Benjamin, 161, 186
Freud, Sigmund, 112
frogs, decisions made by, 197
future tense, in goal-crafting, 183–184

games
    customer care payoff and, 57
    for remembering names, 87
    sales and, 78
Gillespie, Dizzy, 163
gluttony, as Deadly Sin, 117
goal-crafting. *See also* commitment; goals
    achievement dates in, 186–187
    defined, 179
    detail and measurability in, 184–185
    personal progress connecting with, 182
    positive language in, 185–186
    present tense in, 183–184
    role of, 179
    self-assessment, 193

something versus nothing in, 171–174
    writing and visualizing in, 181–182
goals. *See also* goal-crafting
    advertising benefits of, 191–192
    Big PHAT Goals program, 97–101
    defined, 179
    in delegating, 148
    financial, 140
    persistence in achieving, 195–199
    personal and organizational, 41–43
    reassessing, 198–199
    as stepping stones, 24
Goldwyn, Samuel, 85
greed, as Deadly Sin, 117
Grove, Andrew S., 44
Gruen, Father Anselm, 37
Guthrie, Woody, 159

habits, bad, and customer care, 61
Han, Inlark, 67–68. *See also* Donut Man
Han, Jaeyoung, 67
Han, Seongmee, 67
Han, Yoon, 67–68
Harper, Ben, 127
Harris, Sydney, 129
Healthy Balance, 121. *See also* balance
Hopkins, Tom, 52
Horace, 151
How to Win Friends and Influence People (Carnegie), 36–37
human side of change management, 37
humility, as Holy Virtue, 117
humor, as stress defense, 138–139
Hyder, Shama, 26

Iacocca, Lee, 146
IMHO (In My Humble Opinion), 122
incentives. *See* awards; prestige
influence, using positive, 36
information overload, 123
Insta-Progress, 191
internalization, achieving balance, 124–126
journaling, in time management, 152
joy, and motivation, 64–65.
    See also pleasure
Juran, Joseph M., 150

kindness, as Holy Virtue, 117
knowledge
    finding information and, 166–167
    from lifelong learning, 162
    power from, 104
    procrastination and, 158
    questions as source of, 75

leadership, pain and, 94.
    See also Progress Leadership
learning, lifelong, 162.
    See also knowledge
Lee, Ivy, 145, 146
leg up, 86
Lewis, C.S., 27
liberality, as Holy Virtue, 117
The Life and Death of King John (Shakespeare), 30
Lindsay, Ella, 85, 203
Lindsay, Jerry Dean, Sr., 165
Lindsay, Sofia, 85, 203
listening, active, 77–78
The Little Engine That Could (Piper), 203–205
"live and help progress" philosophy, 33
logotherapy.
    See also Frankl, Viktor; power
    introduction to, 48–49
    origin of, 107–109, 112
    philosophy behind, 107
    steps to progress in, 109–111
London, University of, 129
lovely thoughts, against stress, 136
Lubbock, John, 149
Lucifer, 115
lust, as Deadly Sin, 117

Madwed, Sidney, 53
Mandino, Og, 52
Man's Search for Meaning (Frankl), 108–109
Martin, Daren, 146
mastermind groups, 167.
    See also teams, goals of

Maxwell, John, 52
measurement, progress to goals, 184–185
Michelangelo, 187
Monk, Thelonious, 163
Morrison, Jim, 93
motivation
    defined, 30
    joy and, 64–65
    opportunities to provide, 29
    pain as, 94
    responsibility for, 30
motivational speakers, 29
motives, defined, 30
movement, forward, 31–32
music, bop, 162–163

name game, 87. *See also* prestige
negativity, in goal-crafting, 185
networking CODE, 151.
    See also Cracking the Networking CODE (Lindsay)
"next big thing" world, 26
Nietzsche, Frederick, 32
no, saying yes to, 137
Norman, Jessye, 126
Not So Cruddy Service: 7 Habits of Barely Tolerable Service Professionals, 58, 61
nothing, impossibility of doing, 171–174
nutrition, stress management and, 141

omphaloskepsis, 125
organization, respect for, 78–79.
    See also time management
organizations
    in change management, 37
    culture of, 11–12, 64–65
    employees partnering with, 41–43, 44

Pace, Danzae, 133
pain avoidance. *See also* drill sergeant
    assessing promise of, 102
    balancing need for, 93–96
    choices and, 173
    setting goals for, 97–101

Pain leadership and parenting, 94
Pan, Peter, 136
paradoxical intent technique, 141
Parameters of Progress
   defining, 175–177
   discovering others', 34, 75, 77, 80
parents, motivation techniques of, 94
Pareto, Vilfredo, 150
Pareto Principle, 150
Parker, Charlie, 163
partnering, of employees and
   organizations, 41–43, 44
past, dwelling on, 157–158
patience, as Holy Virtue, 117
peace of mind. *See also* customer care
   assessing promise of, 62
   benefits of, 53–54
   from choices made, 173
Penney, J.C., 41
perfection, expecting, 157, 198
persistence, in achieving
   goals, 195–199, 201
perspective, positive, 185–186, 203–205
Peters, Tom, 52
PHAT goals.
   See Big PHAT Goals program
Piper, Wally, *The Little Engine*
   That Could, 203–205
Pirandello, Luigi, 184
planners, how to use, 147.
   See also time management
planning, goals without, 195–196
Plato, 157
pleasure
   assessing promise of, 69
   benefits of, 63–66
   from choices made, 173, 174
   from customer service, 17
   (*see also* Donut Man)
Pope, Alexander, 26
positive perspective, 185–186, 203–205
power. *See also* logotherapy
   assessing promise of, 113
   from choices made, 173
   sources of, 103–105

regret
   defined, 171–172
   self-discipline versus, 95, 205
relationships
   importance of building, 80
   information source on, 36
   time management and, 151
repetition, role of, 204
reward and recognition.
   See awards; prestige
Roach, Max, 163
Robbins, Tony, 52
Rogers, Will, 165
rolling, 165–167.
   See also Stop, BOP, and Roll
Ruskin, John, 116

Saint-Exupéry, Antoine de, 35
sales professionals, 20, 42, 79
Satan, 115
Say Yes to Life in Spite of Everything:
   A Psychologist Experiences the
   Concentration Camp
   (Frankl), 108–109
schedules, setting realistic, 147–148
Schwab, Charles, 145
Seinfeld, Jerry, 171
self-assessment
   goal-crafting, 193
   Progress Agents, 44
   Stop, BOP, and Roll, 168
   stress, 133
   time management, 144
self-discipline, versus regret, 95, 205
self-management, 78–79.
   See also time management
Seneca, Lucius Annaeus, 181
Seven Deadly Sins, 115, 117
Seven Holy Virtues, 117
Seven Wonders of the Ancient World, 177
7 Wonders of the World (NEW), 177
Shakespeare, William, 26
   The Life and Death of King John, 30
Sins, Seven Deadly, 115, 117

Six Ps of Progress.
    See also pain avoidance;
    peace of mind; pleasure; power;
    prestige; profit
  in achieving balance, 123, 125
  choices & reaching, 172–174, 189–191
  learning versus executing, 20, 21
  logotherapy link to, 48–49
  pride and, 115–117
  projected consequences driving, 47
  purpose and, 116
  regret and, 172
  taking action to feel, 50–52
sleep, as stress defense, 140–141
sloth, as Deadly Sin, 117
smiling, during phone calls, 63
Someday Is Not a Day of the Week
    (Brennan-Nelson), 186, 187
Sonny Donuts, 67–68
Southwest Airlines Co., 11–12, 64–65
Spinoza, Baruch, 115
Staubach, Roger, 122
Stein, Gertrude, 19
Stendhal, 66
Stop, BOP, and Roll
  expecting perfection and, 157
  focusing on possibilities in, 161–163
  forward focus in, 157–158
  inevitability of change and, 155
  procrastination in, 158
  self-assessment, 168
  taking action in, 165–167
  wanting versus feeling in, 159
stopping, 157–159.
    See also Stop, BOP, and Roll
stress
  affirmations against, 136
  asking for help with, 142
  choices in reacting to, 132
  debt contributing to, 140
  deep breathing to combat, 138
  everyday causes of, 131
  exercise and, 139
  flexibility in fighting, 142
  humor as defense against, 138–139
  internalizing, 130–131
  as a killer, 129–130
  nutrition and, 141
  saying no and, 137
  self-assessment, 133
  sleep related to, 140–141
  YOU time and, 135
structure, for BAMs, 78–79.
    See also time management
success, versus progress, 23
Suess, Dr., 125
Swiss Family Robinson, 15

Take Time for Progress journals, 152
teams, goals of, 42, 182.
    See also mastermind groups
telephone calls, smiling during, 63
Tennyson, Alfred, 26
thirst, for progress, 75
Thoreau, Henry David, 166
time, spent on stress versus progress, 130.
    See also achievement dates
time management
  business relationships and, 151
  delegating in, 148–149
  efficiency versus effectiveness, 149–150
  goals versus fleeting interests in, 143
  progress blocks in, 151
  progress clocks in, 152
  realistic schedules in, 147–148
  respect for, 78–79
  saying yes to no in, 137
  self-assessment, 144
  starting projects in, 151
  taking time to do things right in, 152
  To-Do Lists in, 145–147, 149
  using planners in, 147
To-Do Lists, 145–147, 149
training, in delegating, 148
trust, as relationship basis, 33
Twain, Mark, 196, 200, 202
Twitter, 26
Two Step System for Progress, 166
Tzu, Sun, 183

Umbrella Man. *See* Donut Man
University of London, 129

upper hand, 72

vacation, ground rules for, 135
value, versus price, 82
verb tense, in goal-crafting, 183–184
Viktor Frankl Institute of Logotherapy, 48
Virtues, Seven Holy, 117
visualization, of goals, 181–182
Vital few and trivial many principle, 150

Waitley, Denis, 52, 72
Walters, Dottie, 73
Walton, Sam, 56
wants, versus feelings, 159
Weber, Julie, 11–12
West, Mae, 143
wrath, as Deadly Sin, 117
writing, of goals, 181–182

Yale Study of Goals, 181
yes, saying no to, 137
YOU time, 135
Youngberg, Carl, 122

zest. *See* pleasure
Ziglar, Zig, 51, 52

About the Author

An authority on harnessing human potential and creating authentic business growth, Dean Lindsay is an engaging and sought-after business consultant and speaker. He is an active member of the Viktor Frankl Institute of Logotherapy and the American Society of Training and Development. Dean has been spotlighted as an Outstanding Speaker by the International Association of Speakers Bureaus and recognized as a "Sales-and-Networking Guru" by the *Dallas Business Journal*.

Dean has served as Guest Lecturer for UCLA and University of Dallas MBA programs, as well as at the International Customer Management Institute. He is a featured contributor to a wide variety of business publications, including: *Executive Travel*, *Sales and Service Excellence*, *Networking Times*, the American Management Association's *Moving Ahead* magazine, and *Selling Power Live*. His first book, *Cracking the Networking CODE: 4 Steps to Priceless Business Relationships*, is recommended reading by the United Professional Sales Association and *Profit* magazine.

A *cum laude* graduate of the University of North Texas, Dean has served on the Executive Advisory Board for UNT's Marketing and Logistics Department and on the Board of Directors for UNT's Alumni Association. Dean is an avid runner and has completed the Stockholm Marathon in Stockholm, Sweden, and the Motorola Marathon, in Austin, Texas. Dean, his wife Lena, and their two strong and wonderfully nutty daughters, Sofia and Ella, live in the Dallas/Fort Worth Metroplex.

Contact Dean at: Dean@DeanLindsay.com.
He would be jazzed to hear from you.

To inquire into Dean Lindsay's consulting and speaking services or for the latest information on *The Progress Challenge* training materials and customized educational programs: Log on to www.DeanLindsay.com

Contact the Author at: Dean@DeanLindsay.com
214-457-5656

Also from Dean Lindsay

Cracking the Networking CODE:
4 Steps to Priceless Business Relationships

Recommended Reading by the
United Professional Sales Association
& Profit magazine

"Perhaps the most powerful way to leverage and multiply your talent and ability is by expanding your personal and business network. **This book shows you how**."
-- *Brian Tracy*
Author, Getting Rich Your Own Way

Copies of Cracking the Networking CODE are available at DeanLindsay.com, Amazon.com and book seller nationwide.